Is Pollution Making You Fat?

Stop Toxins from Creating Fat

Book One of the Lose Weight and Regain Health Series

Dr. Dale Heil

The Lose Weight and Regain Health Series in Order:

Is Pollution Making You Fat? Stop Toxins from Creating Fat

The Psychology Behind Eating: Scientifically Proven Mind Games to Lose Weight and Keep It Off

Foods Making You Fat, Unhealthy, and Unhappy: Your Personal Roadmap to Fix Problems Doctors Cannot

Arthritis, Pain Syndromes, and Feeling Older Than You Should: Your Personalized Path to Stop Pain

Medical Disclaimer

The author does not guarantee any products or recommendations in this book will provide you with the same benefits other people have achieved. You should seek a doctor and do your own research to determine if any of the products or recommendations made by the author in this book will work for you.

While the author has made every effort to provide accurate product names and other information available at time of publication, neither the author nor the publisher assumes responsibility for errors or changes occurring after publication. Additionally, the author has no control over products or websites associated with the products listed in this book or the content of those websites.

This book is sold with the understanding that neither the author nor the publisher is engaged in rendering any legal, accounting, financial, medical, employment, or any other professional advice. If legal, accounting, financial, medical, employment, or any other professional advice is required, the services of a competent professional in those areas should be sought by you. The author and publisher shall have neither liability or responsibility to any person, company, or entity with respect to any loss or damage caused either directly or indirectly by the concepts, ideas, products, information, or suggestions presented in this book. By reading this book, you agree to be bound by the statements above.

CONTENTS

Overview

This is the first book to show how environmental pollution and toxins create vicious cycles of fat production and how to fix this situation.

Do you ever wonder why most people are fat? And why it is so difficult to lose weight and keep it off? This is perplexing when you consider we all eat different foods in varying amounts. The answer is because we all share the same environment. It is the pollution and toxins surrounding us that is making most people carry more fat than they want to.

The chapter on estrogen dominance as a major source of fat production should be particularly interesting to women. But as you will learn, estrogen dominance caused by environmental pollutants affects men as well. Estrogen is often thought of as strictly a female hormone, so men don't see this as a factor contributing to their weight gain.

Then there is stress and how it is guaranteed to put pounds of fat onto your frame if your body cannot expel the hormones that can and will create unending cycles of fat production. And it will remain unending until you take the proper steps to correct this metabolic abnormality. But don't worry, you will learn about that in due time.

Among the tens of thousands of diet books littering bookshelves around the world, none have shown long-term effectiveness. Why would that be? It's because they did not address the actual cause of the phenomenal rise in obesity occurring around the globe. But now, the decades-old techniques of alternative healthcare providers to foster long-term weight loss and health improvements are being made available to the public. And you're reading it!

Chapter Two

Losing Weight and Gaining Health

One should eat to live, not live to eat.

- Moliere

You're fat and you're unhappy about it. Good. Otherwise, you're reading the wrong book.

Don't worry, you are about to discover how to change your life in ways you never dreamed possible.

If you're reading this book, you probably aren't happy with your body and need the correct information to help you get it into shape. This is the knowledge you have sought for a long time, and it will be worth the long wait.

The politically correct term "weight problem" does not adequately describe this condition. As a health care practitioner, I prefer to see health-related issues in terms of having a healthy body and proper eating habits or not. Keeping the issue as clear as possible makes things easier to understand. This helps direct people from a state of ill health to improved health by shifting the focus of the debate away from body weight and onto the root of the problem.

Excess weight is just one of the many consequences of unhealthy body functioning. You may not feel bad or sick all the time, though you could be. But what are those unhealthy body functions and why haven't you been told about them before? We'll talk about that, then lay out an easy-to-follow blueprint for you with many options so you can customize your own plan to suit your personal preferences. You will sing the praises of being healthier after you read the down-to-earth approach this book takes regarding health and losing weight.

We will change your thought processes from simply chasing after weight loss to pursuing improved health. Slimming down is just one of the many benefits of increasing the overall health of your body. If you want to be slimmer, get healthier. It's as simple as that.

This book will teach you very simple strategies to be healthier, and because of being healthier, becoming slimmer.

Everything discussed in the following chapters is based on scientific findings and current trends in understanding how your body processes and uses food energy. I will also pull from my almost forty years of clinical practice experience. By working with patients just like yourself for almost four decades. I know what people are willing to do to lose weight and keep it off, and I know why people fail. The information in this book will help you avoid those pitfalls.

Unlike more restrictive weight loss programs, this book takes the unique approach of creating a system that works within parameters you set for yourself to maintain a healthier and therefore slimmer body. In the past, defining these parameters has been difficult. This isn't your fault.

In contemporary society, we are bombarded with confusing and often conflicting dietary advice. "Eat this and don't eat that," doesn't get you any further than saying, "Eat that but don't eat this." It's all backwards and forwards at the same time. No wonder you may be confused.

Many of the weight loss programs circulating around our world are little more than philosophies of deprivation. By basing our discussion on scientific findings and the actual needs of your body, you will be able to sort the junk dietary ideas from the facts. There is some real rubbish out there, and to make matters worse, much of it is solidly entrenched in medical dogma. To complicate matters, the popular media latches onto a select segment of this dogma and blows its importance (and often its validity) out of proportion. That certainly does not help clarify the subject at all.

One of the most important aspects of any "diet" is it must be realistic. Ask yourself, "How acceptable is this way of eating for myself and my lifestyle?" But the truer test comes from asking, "Can I do this for the rest of my life? Or will I just fall back into my old habits and put all the weight back on?"

This book will show you how to establish a healthy lifestyle for yourself. The next book in this series, The *Psychology Behind Eating: Scientifically Proven Mind Games to Lose Weight and Keep It Off*, will show you a stress-free way to use psychology to make it easy.

Since I mentioned the second book in this book series, let me explain how I organized this information. The second book, as I mentioned, is the psychology book. That book is necessary because our mind dictates how successful we will be losing weight and then keeping it off.

Why lose all that weight just to put it all back on again? And maybe add a few pounds just for good measure? It's what usually happens with people's weight loss efforts, and I wrote this book to avoid that from happening to you.

The third book of the series is entitled *Foods Making You Fat, Unhealthy, and Unhappy: Your Personal Roadmap to Fix Problems Doctors Cannot*. If your goal is only to lose weight and keep it off, the first two books are enough for you. I wrote this third book for people who want to be as healthy as they can be, or those who have terrible health problems they want to reduce or even eliminate.

The fourth book of the series is for people who have very serious health issues that are gravely affecting their lives. It is called *Arthritis, Pain Syndromes, and Feeling Older Than You Should: Your Personalized Path to Stop Pain*.

Each of these books takes the reader further into determining which foods they should eat, and which ones are detrimental to their health. I wrote them in a series because everyone may not want to follow the process to the end because they are happy stopping somewhere along the way. By setting this book series up in this manner, readers can get the results they crave and stop when they want to.

Because extreme diets are not only impractical but also impossible to stick to for years, they are doomed to fail you. The simple changes we will discuss in this book are far from extreme. Then these concepts will be reinforced with physiological and psychological reasoning you can use to prove their worth to yourself. More so than any other diet you've ever tried, this program will last a lifetime.

Oh yeah! The changes recommended in this book will also keep you alive and happy for a long time, assuming you don't get hit by a bus or some other disastrous calamity. This is a good point to remember.

Chapter Three

Why "Diets" Just Don't Work

This is most likely not the first book of this type you've gotten information from. We have all been on the "Diet Roller-Coaster" where you lose weight only to put it all back on… and most likely add a few extra pounds.

The reason for this is simple. Most diets only promote weight loss and are much too radical in their dietary restrictions.

The Pritikin and Ornish diets are at one end of the spectrum and they espouse a vegetarian diet with high carbohydrate intake. On the other end of the spectrum are the Atkins and Protein Power diets. They suggest massive meat and other high-protein food consumption. Others, like the Ketogenic Diet, suggest high fat consumption with low carbohydrate intake.

These diets, when used for weight loss, are much too restrictive to follow for a lifetime even though they make you lose weight. They also deprive your body of essential nutrient intake for extended periods of time. These are the important nutrients you need for basic cognitive and metabolic functions. When stated like this, these diets don't sound very healthy, do they?

You wouldn't stop drinking water for a month if it meant losing a pound or two, would you? Well, that makes as much sense as some diets you see being hyped in the popular media. Not to mention that you may not survive three days if you deprived yourself of water, so don't do that.

Many of the people who used these weight loss diets and liked them at the time are still suffering from unhealthy waistlines. If you are one of them, that's why you're reading this book.

Yes. I know. Some people use popular weight loss diets and are thrilled with them. But if they are truthful with themselves, and after using them for a while, they realize these approaches to eating do not meet all their nutritional or satisfaction needs. Maybe there are only certain parts of those diets that just don't sit well with them. Or cravings for the foods they had to give up become too great and they find themselves back where they started. Except now they feel like a failure. They did not fail. The diet failed them.

The scenario mentioned above (lose weight, then gain it back plus a few extra pounds) is exactly what happened to me when I lost forty pounds on the Atkin's Diet many years ago. It is also what led me to the eye-opening discovery about why we cannot keep the weight off after putting so much willpower and effort into losing it. I found the "missing link," if you will.

While on Atkin's, I maintained my lower weight for two years, but then the inevitable happened.

Because of the restricted food choices of the Atkin's Diet (and most other weight loss diets as well) I succumbed to the temptation to add forbidden foods back into my meals. Not only did I gain back the forty pounds I had lost, putting the weight back on, but I also put on an additional five pounds for good measure. That was not good.

As a clinician, I was used to observing physical changes in other people, but it shocked me when I noticed I'd gained two pounds after eating a small, six-ounce ice cream cone! It was an eye-opening experience because that small ice cream cone did not have the caloric content to account for the weight gain that followed.

At two pounds per ice cream cone, I imagined myself becoming obese within a few years unless I maintained a totally carb-free diet!

Who knew one ice cream cone could cause such an emotionally devastating experience? And trust me, I was devastated.

I had found early in my Atkin's experience that half of the foods allowed on the Atkin's diet would knock me out of ketosis and stop my weight loss. While the incident involving the ice cream cone struck me as odd, I accepted the sugary ice cream as the culprit in my weight gain. I had not otherwise cheated on my diet and had no other explanation of how such a thing could happen. Besides, while on the Atkin's diet I was losing weight, feeling great, and an ultrasound study of my carotid arteries showed them to be clear of plaquing. That was all I cared about as I wanted to avoid dying early of arterial and heart disease, which are epidemic occurrences in our modern world.

Ultimately, the Atkins diet failed me. It was only after regaining all the weight I'd lost, a phenomenon you have likely experienced with much dismay, that I began looking for the answer to why these things were happening. Not only did I delve into all the reference books at my disposal, scour the Internet, and search the local libraries for answers, but I also read every diet book that showed promise.

If I had not had this wealth of information available to me, I may never have noticed the simple answer under my nose the entire time. Well, not under my nose. It was more like several inches above my belly button.

It was my liver making me fat!

Chapter Four

All Roads Lead to the Liver

In decades of clinical practice, I have nutritionally supported the liver for patients suffering from allergies, eczema, hemorrhoids, and varicose veins. I was aware of the role the liver plays in the storage of excess food energy as fat. But it took me years of grueling diets and mental anguish to realize just how much this system could be thrown out of whack. When that occurs, fat storage is affected to an outlandish degree. When the information gelled in my mind, it was like a lightning bolt sending shivers throughout my body. I realized how many people this information could help.

Who would believe nutritional support for your organs has such a tremendous impact on how much excess weight you're carrying? Let me tell you about Harry. Yes, of course it's a fictionalized name, but the patient is real.

I met Harry in my first few weeks of private practice almost forty years ago. If I remember correctly, he was only the third patient through my doors when I started practice, which is one reason his story has stood out in my mind all these years.

Harry was well over 350 pounds and was not happy about it. As a matter of fact, I was afraid he would put me out of business. He was so heavy my treatment table creaked and groaned every time he got on it. They made the table of sturdy wood, but it was the only one I had and if it broke under his substantial weight, I wouldn't have had enough money to replace it. The situation worried me so much I began questioning Harry about his eating habits. I reasoned that If I could help him lose weight, then my table (and my career) might be spared.

As it turned out, Harry only ate a piece of toast for breakfast, half of a sandwich with a piece of fruit for lunch, and a salad or bowl of soup for dinner. The sparseness of these meals couldn't be putting all that weight on him. It was a mathematical impossibility.

Harry's situation had me puzzled until he called me for an emergency visit early one Monday morning.

Over the previous weekend, Harry had spent ten hours driving along the interstate highway, after which he noticed tingling sensations in both his hands and feet.

Harry was certain he'd messed up his neck again with all the driving, and who better to see than his chiropractor? However, after talking to him, it became obvious he was suffering from a condition known as Stocking and Glove Paresthesia, which is a classic indicator of diabetes. A subsequent blood test confirmed this was the case.

Harry began taking a nutritional supplement I suggested that is specifically formulated to support the organs involved in diabetes. He responded immediately. Harry's hands and feet stopped tingling, and he began losing weight.

He thought I was a hero, and while I assured him I was not, inside I felt like one. I really did! To have such success so early in my career was very gratifying. And having proof that all the things I'd spent years learning about worked encouraged me to forge ahead when things got rough (which they always do in clinical practice, and at the most unexpected moment).

I urged Harry to attend a diabetes class at a local hospital so they could teach him how to control his condition with dietary changes, which he did, and he began a walking program for exercise. The weight loss was rapid and significant. Harry lost over 100 pounds in a matter of months. Losing that much weight that fast is not a good idea but try telling that to a man who was obese all his life and suddenly he is losing weight like he never could before. He was on a mission, and he would not be deterred.

Does this mean that everyone has a metabolic condition that, if corrected, will cause rapid and permanent weight loss? No, it doesn't. But what it shows us is that when the body receives the nutritional support it needs, combined with a reasonable diet and exercise, the results can be life changing.

It took many more years after this encounter with Harry until I discovered why people could not lose weight and keep excess body fat off, and it was an epiphany. But it would be misleading to claim I discovered this information on my own. Others much smarter than I am performed the research and to them we owe a great deal, though they are far too many to name. I only gathered this information, interpreted it, and put it to practical use.

One bit of information provided by researchers helped a young man who attended my church. This youngster was so large he could not play with other teens his age. He just could not keep up with his peers and his physical endurance was nil.

During services one Sunday, I studied him. Afterwards, I approached his mother, who my wife and I knew well. When the conversation turned to her son, I told her I didn't think her son was fat, but he was retaining large volumes of water. This water retention created the illusion he was obese.

Her reply was that her son ate little, skipping breakfast and only having a small salad for lunch and half of a sandwich for dinner. Does this sound familiar? It is the same scenario as Harry. This information assured me something other than overeating was at work here.

I suggested she give him a specific nutritional supplement that supported the organs and systems responsible for pumping excess fluid out of the interstitial tissues. It worked. As it turned out, it worked too well. The young man's body began pumping out fluid so quickly his mother reduced his intake from the three tablets per day I had suggested to one per day, rationing a half pill at breakfast and the other half at dinner.

His fluid output was so rapid he was wetting his bed three to four times a night. And this was a teenager who had not wet his bed since he was a small child! Even on the reduced levels of the supplement, he lost 40 pounds in a few weeks. Years later, I saw him as a slim, six-foot-two basketball player preparing to head off to college. His response to the nutritional supplement was nothing short of phenomenal.

Does this mean there is a "miracle" pill out there for you? I doubt it. Life's never that easy.

I told you these two success stories not to inspire you to take pills, but to illustrate that proper nutrition can have dramatic effects. Please don't regard these examples as miracles. They are successes brought about by normalizing the body's basic metabolic functions. Now you are going to learn how to normalize your body's basic metabolic functions, so keep reading.

Chapter Five

What This Book Can Do for You

As an obese child, I remember seeing the controversial weight loss debates between Dr. Atkins and Dr. Pritikin. Even at that young age, I was searching for the answer to having a reasonable amount of fat on my body.

The debate between Atkins and Pritikin has never been settled, as both sides have noteworthy successes and substantial shortcomings. I suspect this book will spark similar fireworks in the popular press. So, what can you expect from this book?

In this book, we will explore what research has revealed in the last few years, much of which is truly eye opening. Many of the findings from research done years ago are still valid today. Some of the older research is even more pertinent now that time has passed, and they have learned new things in the intervening years to better support the older findings. Conversely, some of the hard-felt beliefs once popularized as weight loss panaceas have been invalidated by more recent studies. That's the way science works. New things are learned, and old ones are either supported or proven to be false.

In this book, we will explore why it may not matter what eating habits you choose, because if your liver is not functioning properly, you may never lose weight and keep it off.

I can hear the criticisms now. "He's only a chiropractor!" some will say. And that's true, but the medical field, with its researchers and obdurate beliefs, has failed you time and time again. They could not reduce your weight and have exposed you to significant health risks with diets and treatments that do not treat the holistic nature of the weight loss issue. Therefore, is it any wonder that a novel approach and a method from a decidedly different direction is demanded?

They will probably attack me on several fronts because the information we are about to explore is so foreign to all prior discussions regarding weight loss and health the initial reaction will be to dismiss it as "hogwash."

This doesn't bother me because the method outlined in this book works. It is successful in helping people lose weight, and it explains why all the previous diet fads have failed most people who try them. This book will further your understanding of the situation you find yourself in, and it's important you know what is going on with your body.

I am a practitioner, not a researcher, so some of the information I present to you will be vilified as being out of sync with current dietary fads. "Experts" will come out of the woodwork and attempt to disparage this information.

That's OK. Millions of medical personnel didn't understand the principles of this information before I wrote this book, and they won't want to understand it afterward either. But you will benefit by living a healthier, more fulfilling life, and that's all that's important.

Chapter Six

Don't Ask a Doctor to Change Your Oil

Because of the limits of the private practice environment, I have only been able to help a limited number of patients on a face-to-face basis. But through this book, I will help millions of people around the world. And that is what a health care practitioner does. They help people with their healthcare needs regardless of what obstacles stand in the way.

It always tickles me when patients, after I make nutritional recommendations for them, say, "I want to ask my medical doctor first." Medical doctors are great people, and we owe them a great deal for their service and dedication to humankind. However, most medical doctors are far less knowledgeable about nutrition than the public has been led to believe. This is understandable, as nobody wants to advertise chinks in their armor, so to speak.

But the reality of the situation is the typical medical school does not offer an adequate nutritional education to budding medical doctors. Yet, most people who frequent doctors entrust their medical doctor to give them accurate nutritional advice.

According to patient surveys, medical doctors are widely considered as being one of the most credible sources of nutritional information. This is regardless of large amounts of documentation showing deficiencies in the nutritional knowledge of medical doctors.

One study showed a lack of knowledge and expertise about their patients' nutritional needs has resulted in many medical professionals' reluctance to offer nutritional counseling at all.

If your medical doctor has had specialized training in nutrition or functional medicine, great! Consult with them because they know what they are doing and have the educational background to guide you in your quest for improved health. Without that specialized training, they will almost assuredly lead you down a path they are more familiar with, but it may not be very beneficial to you.

If every medical doctor used appropriate nutritional support in treating their patients, the incidence of patients with unhealthy weight problems would not be the fast-growing, health-jeopardizing issue it is today.

Maybe that's why you're still seeking information and are reading this book.

This is slowly changing with some doctors, such as Raymond D. Strand, M. D., who wrote the book, *What Your Doctor Doesn't Know about Nutritional Medicine May Be Killing You*. This is an interesting book that illustrates what I've been saying.

If you are interested in learning more about the how far behind most doctors are in keeping up with these advancements in science, you can go to my website at www.DEHeil.com where I have a list of resources to make it easy for you to find them and to assure you get the correct books.

Most likely, the only advice you've been getting from the so-called experts is to eat less and exercise more. This is great advice, and something I will also advocate... but with a twist that will make it easy and yield results like you have never seen before. Eating less and exercising more by itself won't lead to long-term weight loss and maintenance because your liver won't let you do it.

Not to mention that eating less and exercising more by itself requires too much sacrifice and willpower. You shouldn't have to sacrifice at all if your liver and digestive system are working correctly.

Another reality the public is unaware of is that most of the true nutritional work being done in the United States is being done by health care practitioners other than medical doctors. Shocking, isn't it?

Nurses, Doctors of Chiropractic (D.C.), Doctors of Naturopathic Medicine (N.D.), Certified Nutritionists, Registered Dietitians/Nutritionists, Pharmacists, and some progressive Medical Doctors that sought additional education are carrying the burden of bringing true nutritional counseling to the American public.

The folks who really know their stuff are the Doctors of Naturopathic Medicine, in my humble opinion. Yes, I'm a Doctor of Chiropractic, and my personal nutritionist is a D.C. also, but we both learned most of what we know from naturopathic doctors, and we're still learning from them.

There is a growing subculture of practitioners putting many sick people on the road to recovery when all other therapies have failed them. This is evidenced by the rapid growth of organizations such as the American Functional Medicine Association and the American Academy of Functional Medicine.

This may come as a shock to you, but it's true.

I must state that medical practitioners are highly educated people and serve a vital function in our health care delivery system. They keep you alive until the health-depleting conditions threatening your life are under control.

Unfortunately, being qualified to offer broad-based and accurate nutritional counseling to keep you healthy after saving your life may not be one of their strengths. That leaves you hanging with no guidance about where you can go or what you should do to maintain your health to avoid future health problems. Let's see if we can't change that by giving you a plan to regain your health and shed some weight in the process.

Chapter Seven

Battle Between Nature and the Pharmacy

Most of the health deteriorating conditions facing Americans today results from them not paying attention to their bodily nutritional requirements as determined by nature. To rectify your health situation (and that includes maintaining a healthy amount of body fat), you must give your body what it needs to function. That sounds simple enough, right?

The medical doctors of today too often rely on drugs or surgery alone to keep you alive. Drugs, on their own and taken on a long-term basis, do not address your bodily requirements, which are nutritional. Just like aspirin and other analgesics can provide temporary relief from chronic pain, prescription drugs only superficially tackle the larger health issues you're suffering from.

Not that short-term drug use is inappropriate, quite the contrary. Medicine clearly has its benefits. For example, where would we be without antibiotics? The medical field undoubtedly makes our lives more pleasant and can add years to our lifespan.

Long-term drug use, however, taken without nutritional support, ignores the obvious problems and does not provide patients with the diligent care and the promise of health they deserve.

You may say, "Sure, I've packed on a few pounds, but I still feel fine. At least my hands and feet aren't tingling!" Great, but just because you feel OK doesn't mean you're at your peak performance, and neither does it mean you're free from hidden health problems.

It's important to remember that the deterioration of health is not a rapid process, but rather a viciously slow one. It can take years before the hardships your body has endured begin threatening your health.

Your body has an amazing capacity to compensate for the abuse you wreak on it, and that can, and will, get you into serious trouble in the long run. This is so evident today that much of what people blame on "getting older" is simply the lack of quality nutritional foods they should consume every day. They've learned to accept these physical and mental shortcomings and they shouldn't… nor do they have to.

In life, there are no shortcuts, and like the deterioration of health, recovery is an equally slow process not achieved overnight. Months, if not years, are needed to reverse the effects of an unhealthy lifestyle and return a depleted body to full health. Luckily, that's to full health. You can make significant and noticeable strides toward a healthier body in a much more reasonable time frame.

It's easier to make simple changes to your lifestyle before physical symptoms surface than it is to repair the damage of prolonged neglect and abuse. True health is easy to lose and hard to regain, but with proper guidance and a little self-determination, true health can be relatively easy to maintain.

But just what is true health? True health is when all your organs and systems are operating at the peak of their efficiency. It is a lot more than the mere absence of disease, though this is part of it.

A saying often attributed to Albert Einstein states that, "Insanity is doing the same thing over and over and over again and expecting different results." Yet that is what most people are doing with their health and eating habits.

Most of you reading this book have tried the same diets repeatedly. Losing weight only to regain it. This is insanity as Einstein saw it. The time has come to try something new.

The pleasant irony of the method outlined in this book is that for you to lose weight and keep it off, you are going to forget about dieting and losing weight. Pretty cool, huh?

That's because this is not a "diet book" the way you've probably come to view them. It is a statement of the facts of nature, an easy-to-follow roadmap that will help you see the truth and reach a logical conclusion based on research, common sense, and what works for you. And, of course, this conclusion will lead you to the attainment of a healthier level of weight and improved general health.

You will not concentrate on losing weight. However, you are going to concentrate on a health centered approach that will allow you to be healthier in several ways. In the process, you will get a more desirable physique and a more appropriate body weight, which is the natural progression on the road to regaining your health.

Living healthy or unhealthy. The choice is yours and yours alone. I'm going to show you how, and it's easy if you want to know the truth. You just need to ask yourself, "Am I willing to take responsibility for my health if it will result in a slimmer body?" instead of asking, "What do I need to do to lose weight?"

Weight loss alone does not guarantee improved health. While we're being honest, you should also ask yourself if it's worth it to endure the hassle of a restrictive diet when you're not one bit healthier in the end. You may look nicer in a bathing suit for a short time, but are you truly healthier? A healthier body will make long term weight maintenance a reality.

You can either embrace a healthier, slimmer life or choose to ignore the simple facts and lead an unhealthy, miserable existence. That may sound harsh, but it's always been your choice and yours alone.

Remember that becoming healthier is not just a personal goal. By becoming healthier, you will also serve as a role model for your children. If, by watching you improve your health, your children learn to avoid the plague of having unhealthy eating habits and compromised fitness, you've taught them an invaluable lesson.

Buckle up and get ready for an eye-opening experience. Your life is about to change in an enormous way!

Chapter Eight

Pollution, Fat, and A Possible Solution?

Webster's Deluxe Unabridged Dictionary, Second Edition, defines a pollutant as something that taints, defiles, or contaminates; especially a harmful chemical or waste material discharged into the water or atmosphere. And pollutants may contribute to the unhealthy amount of weight you are carrying.

How can pollution possibly contribute to you carrying more weight than you are comfortable with? Pollution and toxins, when absorbed in quantities that overwhelm the ability of your liver to excrete them, cause several vicious fat-producing cycles to be established.

Your liver is the organ responsible for determining if the food you eat is used to fuel your body immediately or is stored as fat. In later chapters, you will learn exactly how an overworked and overloaded liver contributes to fat production.

The weight loss system we will discuss is about getting healthier and not just about losing weight. Keep that in mind.

Most people want to start on a weight loss program without considering what is causing their body to retain excess fat. They often blame it on overeating or their inability to control themselves around food. Both viewpoints can lead to devastating mental anguish that is incorrect and misleading.

Weight loss diets alone skip the vital first step, which is to get your liver working correctly so it can stop the fat producing effects of pollution. After that, any weight loss program will more efficiently remove excess fat from your body. This may be especially important for children.

Why should we be concerned about children?

Because children are in grave danger of developing serious health damaging conditions at an early age, and these are preventable. Obesity is at epidemic proportions for children in many areas of the world. By establishing a healthy weight in children who are at risk, much suffering, monetary loss, and lost years of life can be avoided.

Obesity can affect us in many ways other than simply how we look. Being overweight may mean you're losing money, possibly a lot of money, and you will continue to do so if you don't get your act together.

Way back in the year 2000, The Surgeon General's "Call to Action to Prevent and Decrease Overweight and Obesity" reported the combined costs of being overweight in the U.S. was more than $117 billion dollars. That was $61 billion dollars in direct health care costs and $56 billion in indirect costs. Those figures are much higher today, but not much else has changed. Obesity is still a huge and costly problem.

So what? You have health insurance to cover any health problems you get from being overweight that will pay for your care, right? Maybe. But you will still have significant out-of-pocket expenses you probably did not budget for. Remember that the deductible and co-pay on health insurance comes directly out of your pocket. There are also out-of-pocket expenses you accrue for over-the-counter medications, the cost for transportation to and from doctor's offices, and lost time at work. You may even find yourself paying someone else to do household maintenance because you are too big or sick to do it yourself. All these expenses add up.

Indirect costs you may never see include the increased health insurance costs to your employer that must be paid on all employees because premiums are based upon the entire group. That's less money your employer has in their grubby little hands to give you a raise the next time you ask.

Wasted money cannot be used for things that may be more important to you. If you can't afford a vacation trip this year it may be because you had to spend your disposable income on problems arising from your deteriorating health.

But the biggest loss you will experience from not improving your health doesn't have a set value. By not lowering your weight, you're losing significant portions of the joy of life. The thrill of living is priceless. Your life is too precious to waste months, weeks, or even days not feeling well enough to live it fully. Getting your weight closer to the normal range will allow you to enjoy the physical and monetary benefits that come with it.

Let's move on to determine if pollution and its effect on your liver may be a contributing factor to your unhealthy weight.

Chapter Nine

Pollution and Weight Gain

Before we get into the nuts-and-bolts of why pollution may cause your unhealthy accumulation of body fat by overloading your liver, let's determine if you even have this problem. We will go into detail later as to exactly how and why pollution causes problems, but for now, let's concentrate on you.

As you review the bodily signs and symptoms listed below, try to evaluate whether you have them, but also if they are frequent occurrences for you or not. Recurring problems need correction. If these problems occur only infrequently, then you may be on the edge of developing an unhealthy situation. If these never occur, then you're OK, for now at least.

The greater the number of these symptoms plaguing you, and the more frequently they occur, the worse off you are. Ask yourself:

Do you often have nausea or vomiting for no good reason?

How about frequent diarrhea or constipation? Or a combination of the two where you can't move your bowels but when you manage to get them moving, you really bust loose.

Do you have a lot of gas in your stomach (under the left side of your rib cage) or in your lower belly, resulting in excessive flatulence (passing of gas)? Does gas in your belly occur shortly after eating? Are certain foods causing these problems more than other foods? Does eating fatty foods make you feel sick?

Is heartburn a problem? If it is present, does it occur either immediately after eating or within two hours of finishing a meal?

In your mind, these digestive signs and symptoms may easily be associated with the liver or gut tube; but how about symptoms that may affect your ears or even your eyes? Do you have itchy ears, either inside or outside the ear canal?

How about ringing in your ears, or hearing loss that is not because of damage from loud noises in your earlier years?

Are frequent earaches, ear infections, or even drainage from your ears a common situation with you?

Do your eyes have dark circles under them or give you tunnel vision (in the absence of glaucoma or other identified eye disorders)? How about having blurred vision, itchy, or watery eyes with or without red, sticky eyelids? Each of these can be a sign or symptom of interest. Make a list of the symptoms that pertain to you because you will need this list later.

While we're in the head area, do you suffer headaches, fainting, dizziness, or pressure inside your head?

How are your emotions? Under control most of the time or not?

As you will see later in the chapter on estrogen (which can affect men and women), these emotional situations may or may not be related to hormones alone. The inability of an overloaded liver to effectively metabolize excess amounts of estrogen or chemicals that mimic the effects of estrogen may be at fault.

Mood swings, anxiety, fear, nervousness, and depression are rampant in our society, and they may all be signs of a dysfunctional liver.

Are you angry or irritable? Do you have a sense of despair? Are you apathetic or sluggish with no energy? If so, you'd better look at an overloaded liver as a possible contributing factor.

Is your memory not what it used to be? It may not just be advancing age or your children that are making you more forgetful. Are you often confused or having problems with concentrating on something that should have your undivided attention? Don't blame something on the wrong reason it is happening. That can lead you down the wrong path resulting in you not getting to the root of the problem.

Is it often difficult to make simple decisions? Are you becoming more uncoordinated in your movements, suffering from slurred speech, or having trouble learning new things? These can also be symptoms of a stroke, so it is good to have a thorough examination by your medical doctor or a neurologist. Don't just assume an overloaded liver is causing all these symptoms.

Has your energy, vim, and vigor gone away? Has all the iron in your blood turned into lead in your bottom?

Sorry. I couldn't resist throwing a little humor into this long list of boring symptoms to lighten things up a bit.

Remember that your skin is a secondary excretory organ. If your liver cannot metabolize the toxins in your bloodstream, your skin will try to excrete them. While this is an adaptive mechanism established by your body to be used in emergencies, your skin can get damaged in the process, so it is not a viable long-term solution.

So, what types of skin disorders signal a liver overloaded with toxins? Acne, rashes (including conditions like eczema), dry skin, hives, flushed skin, or excessive sweating may all be signs of the skin becoming involved in an excretory activity it really is not fully equipped to perform.

Your mucous membranes also may be affected by liver congestion. This could cause something as innocuous as a stuffy nose, hay fever, sinus problems, sneezing attacks, or excessive mucus production in your nose.

Your throat may often feel dry. Are you always having a chronic cough, with or without gagging, and feel the need to clear your throat constantly? The frequent appearance of canker sores in your throat and mouth, which may also be accompanied by swollen or discolored gums, could be indications of a congested liver. Who would have ever thought that all these seemingly unrelated problems could have a common cause?

The lungs can try throwing off toxins so they may begin giving you shortness of breath, chest congestion, asthma, or bronchitis type symptoms. All these types of symptoms may lead to breathing difficulties, and that's dangerous, so make sure you let your doctor know.

Carrying around toxins in your bloodstream may cause fatigue, hyperactivity, restlessness, insomnia, or even being startled awake from a deep sleep.

What? You thought an overloaded liver would only affect you during the day? Oh, no. Waking at 3 a.m. every night may be from your liver becoming active... at least according to acupuncture theory. I have had enough experience with this phenomenon to consider the liver immediately as the culprit.

An overloaded liver affects other major organs, such as the heart that results in skipped heartbeats, rapid heartbeats, and even chest pains. It can also affect the immune system with an increased frequency of minor illnesses like head colds and stomach flu. The genitalia and urinary tracts are prime candidates for involvement with a congested liver. Frequent or urgent urination, or even a leaky bladder, may be a sign of sluggish liver involvement.

Naturally, the muscles and joints are often involved because they seem to react every time the immune system is compromised. Just like the flu, symptoms may include joint pain, muscle pain, recurring backaches, or feelings of "tired" or "weak" muscles with no physical activity being performed. The liver can be a precipitating factor.

Then there's the weight problem, which is probably the topic you're most interested in hearing about. Everything from binge eating to compulsive eating can be traced to an overloaded liver. That includes craving certain foods, water retention, or excess weight gain.

What about your inability to handle caffeine since you've gotten older? The liver metabolizes caffeine to get it out of your body, and it is usually very efficient at this job. But if your liver is not removing it from your bloodstream quickly and efficiently, caffeine just keeps circulating, keeping you on edge for long periods of time or disturbing your sleep at night. That's why you could handle it when you were younger (when your liver was not as overloaded with toxins) but can't now (after your liver is overloaded). Age may have nothing to do with it.

That's a lot of things that can cause noticeable symptoms caused by an overloaded liver. Quite a few very common things, wouldn't you say? Maybe liver overload is much more common than you ever imagined? And that's if you even knew such a condition as an overloaded liver existed.

To understand why these symptoms occur, you need to understand how your liver works. Let's take a few minutes and review what takes place in the liver.

How Your Liver Works

Everyone wants to know how pollution is overloading their liver and making them fat and what they can do about it. And they want to know now!

Well, before we can get to the good stuff, a basic understanding of how your liver affects your general health and weight is in order.

Your liver is a hard-working organ performing a multitude of functions essential to life. It is a chemical factory because it makes many substances, including blood glucose, which is made from sugars that were stored in the liver as glycogen. Glucose is manufactured and released into the bloodstream when needed. For example, when a person is sleeping but not eating their blood sugar levels must be maintained to fuel and maintain their bodily functions, and their liver takes care of that task.

Inside your liver, cholesterol is used to make bile, which aids in digestion. The cholesterol made by the liver is also needed to make important hormones such as estrogen, testosterone, and adrenal hormones. Cholesterol is also a vital component of every cell membrane, so your body needs lots of it.

Even removing damaged cells and rebuilding new ones is associated with your liver when it makes bilirubin to aid in breaking down old or damaged red blood cells. There is some evidence that higher levels of bilirubin can help reduce the incidence of cardiovascular disease. How does it accomplish this? It acts as an antioxidant, reducing the damage caused by free radicals as they float through the bloodstream. So, the functions of your liver may affect other organs and bodily systems.

Your liver also makes albumin, which is a protein that is needed to maintain fluid pressure in the bloodstream. Other proteins are created that make up the clotting factors of blood to stop bleeding. As you can see, your liver is involved in an array of functions occurring throughout your entire body.

Your liver is a bit like a trapeze artist. It balances nutrients absorbed from food to maintain homeostasis (the healthy equilibrium of bodily systems) while excreting waste to rid your body of toxins. At least it should if it is operating correctly.

When sub-optimal functioning of your liver occurs, it can cause many problems and symptoms within your body. While discussing the phenomenon of a sub-optimally functioning liver, we will call it an "overloaded" liver for brevity and ease of understanding.

Your liver plays a major role in the detoxification of drugs and chemicals. Since it is placed strategically between your intestines and the rest of your body, it filters bacteria entering the bloodstream through your gut. This keeps the invaders from being carried throughout your body wreaking havoc on your other organs, glands, and tissues.

Let's take a quick look at each of the various jobs your liver performs.

While maintaining homeostasis, your liver controls blood sugar, proteins, fats, and cholesterol levels while removing excess hormones such as estrogen and cortisol from the bloodstream (which we will discuss as these can cause fat being deposited where you don't it to be). It also stores essential vitamins, including fat-soluble vitamins like A, D, K, and E.

The liver plays a major role in the conversion of excess blood sugar (glucose) into glycogen, which is stored in muscle and the liver itself. When needed for energy, the liver extracts and converts stored glycogen back into glucose for your body to use as energy. By your liver being able to instantaneously perform a glycogen-to-glucose conversion, it can maintain a blood glucose balance essential to normal brain function. The importance of this one function is immeasurable since glucose is the only fuel source for your brain.

Specific functions of the liver of particular interest in our discussion concerning weight loss are the processes of purification, transformation, and clearance of toxic materials from the body. Collectively, these processes are known as detoxification.

There are two phases to the detoxification process during which the liver breaks down harmful compounds that must be excreted from the body. For this excretion, or toxic eviction as it is sometimes called, to take place, the harmful chemicals must be converted, or "conjugated," into a water-soluble form. Only when the toxins are water soluble can they pass from the body in the urine.

Another avenue for chemical removal is the excretion of toxins via bile, where they are dumped into the intestines and expelled from the body in feces.

Are you falling asleep yet? Stay with me. This stuff is important even though it may be boring to learn. You must know what is going on, so you do not fall back into only thinking in terms of simply losing weight. There are tremendous health benefits to be realized if you do what your body needs to be done.

Phase I of the detoxification process occurs when the toxins are changed into other chemicals. These altered chemicals are also known as intermediate chemicals or intermediate metabolites. After they are made, they move to the second stage, known as Phase II, where they are conjugated (converted) into their final form so they can be gotten rid of.

The inability of the liver to perform Phase I or Phase II of the detoxification process efficiently results in a condition known as "overloaded" liver. That's the main function of the liver we are interested in for warding off weight gain.

There are two reasons the liver becomes overloaded. The first occurs when the sheer volume of toxins coming into the body overwhelms the liver's ability to process them all. The second occurs when there are not enough enzymes and other essential nutrients in the diet. Without enough enzymes and/or essential nutrients being available to the liver, it cannot process the quantity of toxins it must excrete. When either of these problems occur, the entire process backs up like a clogged sewer.

Pay close attention now. This is stuff you must understand. Also, you must be serious about making the changes necessary so your body will allow you to lose weight.

Not only does an overloaded liver contribute to a person packing on pounds of fat, but it can lead to much more serious health problems. The ability, or inability, of an individual to excrete toxins may be why some people develop serious diseases like cancer while others, when exposed to the same environmental levels of carcinogens, do not. Toxins lingering in the body have a longer time to change the genetic make-up of the cells, resulting in cancer formation.

Understanding the importance of the liver's functions, and the degree to which it is performing those functions, allows healthcare providers to apply programs that will aid in recovery from diseases in which liver functioning plays a vital role. For instance, some research suggests that impaired liver detoxification is implicated in health conditions such as chronic fatigue syndrome, fibromyalgia, and pancreatitis. If you suffer from these conditions, and your doctor does not look toward the liver as to why you're suffering from them, you may miss out on finding a solution to your dilemma.

When exposure to chemicals occurs, the elevated levels of them in the bloodstream demand the liver increase Phase I activity to rid the toxins from the body. After Phase I makes the intermediate chemicals, Phase II must work overtime to handle the sudden increase.

However, an unhealthy liver won't be able to conjugate the huge amounts of intermediary chemicals being produced. Failure of Phase II conjugation to turn the intermediary chemicals into water-soluble compounds results in a toxic chemical build-up.

Both phases of liver detoxification must run at full speed to avoid having non-excreted toxins linger in the body, where the longer they remain, the more damage they can do. Even a slight decrease in liver detoxification efficiency can lead to an "overloaded" liver where it cannot keep up with the demands placed upon it.

There are other problems that can arise that may or may not be directly related to the amount of toxins your body must deal with. For instance, your liver also excretes excess hormones such as estrogen and cortisol. These are very important to our discussion. These hormones, when in excess, create and trap fat within your body.

If your liver cannot excrete the excess hormones responsible for fat retention, you are on the road to forming and keeping an unhealthy accumulation of body fat. Raised levels of these hormones almost guarantee fat storage.

Liver conditions may inhibit the detoxification process. Ironically, the intermediary chemicals created in Phase I may be more toxic than the substances they started out as. This is a major problem if Phase II cannot keep up and conjugate them into compounds that can be excreted as soon as possible.

Why does your body create intermediary chemicals in the first place if they are more harmful than the original toxins? In most cases, it is easier for your body to convert the intermediary chemical into a water-soluble form. So, it temporarily creates a stronger poison that's easier to manipulate. In doing so, your body is operating under the expectation that these intermediary chemicals will be immediately converted and excreted.

Your body doesn't expect these harmful chemicals to hang around any longer than necessary. Unfortunately, if your liver is overloaded because Phase II cannot keep up, this is exactly what happens.

Intermediary chemicals are not a problem if Phase II is ready to render them harmless immediately. The big question is whether Phase II is ready and able to perform its job.

Are you seeing how your liver, if it is impaired, even to a small degree, may contribute to you being unable to lose excess fat? Think of your liver in terms of the snowball effect. If it falls a little behind in its operations, a problem that started out small can become larger when more and more toxins build up. Make sense? Good! Now pay attention because it gets better.

Also affecting your liver's ability to function in this detoxifying capacity is the exposure to various chemicals or toxins you consume on purpose. This includes alcohol and many prescription drugs. As is often the case with an overloaded liver, prescription drug dosages may need to be reduced or, sometimes, discontinued all together if the liver cannot metabolize and excrete toxic residues.

Drug exposure, or exposure to other toxins, may affect the ability of the liver to function correctly, resulting in anything from a mild liver dysfunction up to a life-threatening situation.

Another important function of the liver, which we already touched upon briefly, is to synthesize (manufacture) cholesterol. Cholesterol is a type of lipid (think of it as a type of fat), found in cell membranes. It is also a major constituent of the insulation around your nerves. This insulation prevents your nerves from "shorting out." That's important!

Cholesterol is vital to the functioning of the body. When you don't consume enough cholesterol from food sources every day, your liver will manufacture cholesterol from other fats to make up for the lack. This ensures a ready supply is available to insulate your entire nervous system.

If you eat a lot of cholesterol in a single day, a healthy liver will respond by manufacturing less cholesterol. Your liver makes sure the daily-required level of cholesterol is available to your body despite fluctuations and inconsistencies in your diet. And let's be honest, what you eat varies from day to day.

As great as your liver is, an overload of environmental pollutants and chemicals (either man-made, those that occur in nature, or those manufactured by your body itself) can make the liver sluggish, overload it, and reduce its ability to safeguard your body from harmful compounds.

Don't be confused. Having an overloaded liver does not mean your liver is diseased. It's simply not functioning up to its full potential. It's possible to have an overloaded liver showing no signs of liver damage, which is what the usual blood tests for liver disease reveal. Blood tests will show normal liver enzymes even if your liver is overloaded and unable to perform its normal excretory functions.

The usual medical tests for liver disease look for excess liver enzymes in the blood that rise to abnormally high levels when liver cells rupture. This occurs only if the liver is truly diseased. However, normal liver enzyme levels will be found in the blood with early-stage liver overload. Overload refers only to the inability of the liver to perform its detoxification functions, but not to the health or integrity of the liver itself.

The reduced liver operating capacity found in the overloaded liver can lead to many physical symptoms you would never consider as being related to the liver. These symptoms may include things like fatigue that is not associated with physical activity, out-of-control anger (maybe "Road Rage" and other mood swings could be an example of this?), hormonal imbalances including pre-menstrual syndrome (PMS), fibromyalgia and a whole gamut of other aches and pains that evade easy diagnosis. Even high blood pressure may result from this situation.

With high blood pressure, you must work with your medical doctor while on any liver detoxification (also known as liver cleansing or purification) program, which is what we will talk about shortly. This is because your blood pressure may come down as your liver functioning improves. If that occurs, your medication must be appropriately adjusted or discontinued altogether to avoid dropping your blood pressure too low.

If your blood pressure returns to normal after liver detoxification, expect some resistance from your medical doctor in discontinuing the medication as they are taught that once high blood pressure is present, it will always be present. Therefore, they may be reluctant to take you off the medication even if high blood pressure symptoms have subsided.

The confusion here is understandable, as standard medical education and experience supports the "life-time medication" approach for high blood pressure. This line of thinking may change when more people recondition their livers to work at maximal functioning capacity.

Problems previously viewed by healthcare practitioners as permanent and requiring lifelong consumption of prescription drug cocktails may be revealed as temporary conditions resulting from impaired liver performance. If you detoxify your liver and improve its ability to perform its job correctly, you may find that conditions plaguing your health for years disappear.

Be patient and monitor your body, noting any changes that occur after liver detoxification. There may be other symptoms not mentioned that accompany an overloaded liver. Let's review them.

Chapter Eleven

Is Your Liver Overloaded?

Additional chronic symptoms not previously mentioned that may be related to an overloaded liver include, but are not limited to:

- Allergies (Have you ever wondered why allergies are becoming a bigger and bigger epidemic these days?)
- Asthma (another condition reaching epidemic proportions)
- High Cholesterol (again, at epidemic proportions)
- Skin conditions such as eczema (Aaaah, another condition at epidemic levels, right?)
- Blood sugar regulating problems like diabetes and hypoglycemia (Uh, oh. Are you seeing a pattern of epidemics forming here?)
- Headaches
- Bad breath
- Dark circles under the eyes
- Body odor (the type where you still stink even after a shower)
- Nausea
- Diarrhea
- Constipation
- Bloating of the intestinal tract (a very common occurrence, wouldn't you say?)
- Out of control flatulence (no husband jokes, please!)
- Difficulty losing weight
- Difficulty gaining weight (life is strange sometimes, isn't it?)
- Indigestion

- Muscle pain not explained by exertion
- Unexplainable joint pain
- Depression
- Anxiety
- General irritability
- Frequent illness such as colds, flu, sinus infections, etc.
- Sensitivity to chemicals such as cleaning supplies
- Hemorrhoids
- Varicose veins
- Fatigue
- Metallic taste in the mouth
- Pale, pasty skin that looks papery
- Difficulty sleeping
- Mentally dull
- Low libido
- Cravings for certain foods
- Fibromyalgia
- Fluid retention

Having a symptom or combination of symptoms on this list does not mean you have an overloaded liver. There are many causes for all the conditions on this list, but if your liver is causing these symptoms, then all the pills, potions, and lotions in the world will not help you until your liver is functioning properly.

An overloaded liver rarely occurs by itself and is usually accompanied by gut tube malfunction. Soon, under the Leaky Gut Syndrome section, we will discuss how a sick gut will lead to liver overload. You didn't think this would be a straightforward problem with a singular solution, did you? Good, because it's not.

Then there is the situation known as fatty liver. It can occur independently of, or may be related to, a liver overloaded by pollution. Let's explore the condition known as fatty liver first because it is another epidemic plaguing the world's population.

Chapter Twelve

Fatty Liver and Body Fat

A healthy liver has the physical ability to filter the blood to remove toxins, bacteria, viruses, and other debris from the blood. That's its job, to act as the "oil filter" of the body and get all the "crud" that is not supposed to be there out of the system.

However, if the liver accumulates fat within itself the ability of the liver to perform these vital functions plummets. This condition is commonly known as fatty liver.

Please take the time to differentiate in your mind between an "overloaded" liver and a "fatty liver." An overloaded liver cannot efficiently process toxins out of the body because it has too much work to do and not enough of the resources it needs to do it. A fatty liver is where fat cells are deposited inside the liver, reducing the ability of the liver to filter bad stuff out of your blood.

Healthy liver cells detoxify toxins to keep the body functioning properly. Fat cells just sit in the liver doing nothing except taking up valuable space. The fat in the liver physically slows or stops the flow of blood through the liver, further reducing its ability to clear toxins from your body.

To better visualize what a fatty liver is, think of a liver with fat globs accumulating inside the cells of the liver and in the spaces between those cells. This fat accumulation causes the liver to become larger and heavier. It becomes a sack of fat.

Fatty liver is one way your liver can lose the ability to perform its job. The overall effect is the same as an overloaded liver but reduced clearing of toxins is happening for different reasons. Both conditions result in toxins not being removed from your body in a timely manner.

The same type of process occurs in your car's oil filter when it becomes clogged with dirt. However, your car's oil filter can easily be replaced to restore its function. Your liver can't.

The liver processes most fats so a diet that is high in fat, includes high alcohol consumption, or a diet that is poor in nutrients may cause a liver that cannot burn fat correctly or send it out into the bloodstream as it is meant to. Instead, the fat is stored in the cells of the liver and stays there.

Two substances, choline and carnitine, are essential to the proper processing of dietary fat. If your diet is high in fat, both substances may be depleted because they are used up faster than they can be replaced.

Choline is a major component necessary to produce bile. It is bile that processes fats in the gut to get the fat ready for absorption. Bile also carries the metabolized toxins from your liver to the gut tube for excretion. Both steps are very important functions.

If your diet is high in carbohydrates and high in fats, it will promote the conversion of the carbohydrates to triglycerides, further depleting the amount of choline in your body. Eating a lot of carbohydrates and fat sounds like the typical American diet, doesn't it? It's easy to see why such a diet can cause a multitude of problems.

Estrogen (which you will read more about later) also depletes choline. This may be why women have more problems with the gallbladder (where the bile is stored) than do men.

Carnitine, on the other hand, moves fat into the mitochondria. They are the "powerhouse" of the cells where energy is produced for the cells to operate. The mitochondria are where fat is converted to energy for healthy cellular function.

If your diet does not contain enough carnitine, or your body is rapidly depleting it because of the large volume of fat you consume, then fat cannot move into the mitochondria to be burned for energy. That's not too hard to understand, is it?

If the fat in your diet is not being burned for energy, then it must be stored. That's important, because it will be stored in larger quantities and in places you don't want it to be stored.

The bottom line, once again, is that the typical American diet does not supply the nutrients necessary for efficient fat burning. Instead, it promotes fat storage.

For you to lose fat and become healthy, you must supply the nutrients your liver and body need to function correctly. That means consuming foods that promote proper liver functioning.

These are the rules your body plays by. There are no shortcuts or deletions in this game. You either abide by the rules and achieve health, or you don't. It's your choice and your choice alone. Your body doesn't make "deals" just because you want to eat the foods that will harm it.

Obesity can lead to fatty liver. It is now accepted that the non-alcoholic fatty liver (that which is not caused by excessive alcohol consumption) is because of insulin resistance. However, insulin resistance (a condition where blood sugar cannot be used by the body's cells the way it is supposed to be used) is associated with the incidence of obesity. One bad thing just seems to feed off the other to create more problems for you.

Insulin resistance is part of the metabolic syndrome that may become such a large part of the consequences of having unhealthy weight levels. Recent studies, at least in mice, have found that fatty liver correlates with the presence of insulin resistance. Even some human studies have shown that fatty liver appears to be associated with insulin resistance. We need more research to make that determination more definitive.

Obesity has not been specifically implicated in the formation of a fatty liver until recently. But now, at least one study appears to show the contribution obesity makes to the formation of a fatty liver. So, if you've been following this, you can see that obesity can create a situation that then impedes your liver's ability to function correctly. That may lead to more fat being stored instead of being burned. Got that? Good!

Since Type 2 diabetes is also associated with insulin resistance, it is reasonable to think that a fatty liver is part of this triad. A fatty liver may have some predictive value in the appearance of type 2 diabetes as a disease entity.

Fatty liver contributes to fat storage because it inhibits the ability of the liver to detoxify and expel toxins from the body. Since fat creates estrogen (which you will soon learn a lot more about) and estrogen turns around and creates more fat, you soon find yourself in one of the vicious cycles of fat production you do not want to be in.

A fatty liver is nothing to ignore. It is the most common liver disease, not only in the United States, but throughout the world as well. It affects ten to twenty-four percent of the world's population. In the United States alone, it is estimated that over twenty-nine million people suffer from a fatty liver. The alarming part of this statistic is that it is now being found in children.

Of course, these figures may be on the low side. Fatty liver does not present with any symptoms and is usually only diagnosed when a routine liver enzyme test shows elevated levels of liver enzymes circulating in the bloodstream.

One common cause of liver failure necessitating a liver transplant to save the patient's life is a condition called cryptogenic cirrhosis. It is believed that this condition is the late stages of fatty liver. Soon, liver diseases caused by obesity are expected to become the leading cause of liver failure and liver transplant surgery.

I told you this stuff is nothing to mess with!

Chapter Thirteen

Where Do Toxins Come From?

The toxins your liver must deal with are all around you. Let's look at information supplied by the U.S. Environmental Protection Agency to see where these bad things come from.

In a publication entitled "The Inside Story: A Guide to Indoor Air Quality" the EPA outlines some of the worst offenders and identifies where they come from. You may only think of outside pollution from automobiles, factories, or energy-producing plants when considering the source of toxins, but indoor toxins are just as important, if not more important, than the outdoor variety.

We face many assaults from our environment every minute of every day. We inhale exhaust fumes from cars, trucks, and fly in airplanes while breathing re-circulated air. After our commute to our job, we work all day in offices with similarly closed environments. People who work in factories or in the construction trades have their own types of toxins to deal with, which may or may not be worse than what office workers must deal with.

Researchers discovered that toxins were found in bodily tissues in more than half of the people studied. Data such as this suggests that most people are carrying a toxic load in their bodies from long-term exposure. Toxins continue accumulating throughout your lifetime, resulting in large accumulations within your body. Because of this accumulating effect, the amount of toxins found in you may be much greater than environmental concentrations would suggest. Your body is concentrating this stuff.

Since you can't avoid all the environmental toxins you are exposed to, your body must expel them before they can do much harm. This means you must supply your body with the phytonutrients (also known as phytochemicals) your liver must have to flush the toxins out of your system. Phytonutrients are bioactive chemical compounds found in plants that play a major role in ridding your body of toxins and in protecting your tissues from their detrimental effects.

Phytonutrients are very important and only come from plants. Remember that tidbit for later because you must increase your intake of raw vegetables and fresh fruits to supply phytonutrients to keep your liver functioning correctly, and not because they are low in calories to make you lose weight.

Make your body healthier and you lose weight in the process. Isn't that what I said? Phytonutrients from plants are a major component of this scenario, so eat your raw vegetables. Your body will thank you for it.

Here's a real kick in the pants. The air in your home and other buildings you spend time in is more polluted than the outdoor air is in our largest and most industrialized cities.

Here's a second kick in the pants. Most people spend about ninety percent of their time indoors.

Are you ready for the third kick in the pants? The people who are most susceptible to the effects of indoor air pollution such as the ill, the young, and the elderly, are inside most of the time. This is especially true for the folks suffering from heart or arterial disease, or those with breathing problems, who spend most of their time indoors.

So, where do toxins come from?

They come from many sources. Anything that releases gas vapors or puts particles of matter into the air can be a source of indoor air pollution. These types of sources make up a large pool of potential problem areas.

The concentration of pollutants (toxins) increases with reduced airflow through a building, by higher temperatures, or even by higher humidity levels. OK, so these environmental factors may cause a higher concentration of pollutants within your buildings, but how do toxins get inside buildings?

That's easy. You bring them in.

Items like tobacco, gasoline, kerosene, etc. do not have to be burned to emit toxins. Insulation, carpets, paints, furniture finish, and glues from compressed wood products release gases in your home or office building just by sitting there.

Common household items such as cleaning products, personal care products like hair spray, glues you use in your hobbies, and the epoxies you use to maintain your home release toxins. Most common household items release toxic gases. You then inhale these pollutants into your lungs with each breath.

There is no realistic way to escape exposure to toxins in today's world. For instance, a pilot study looking at residential toxin exposure discovered thirty-three different carcinogens (cancer-causing agents) known to cause breast cancer in common household dust. Besides the toxins found in dust, these researchers also found twenty-four different compounds in the air of residences.

Some areas of the United States pose a high risk for the release of radon gas, a major cause of lung cancer. Radon gas emanates from the rock and soil beneath buildings and becomes trapped in sealed homes. It doesn't matter if it's heating or cooling season. Homes are sealed (probably with a sealant that releases toxins into the air!) to prevent the loss of costly temperature-controlled air.

Other areas of the country have pesticides applied to or around building foundations to prevent destruction by termites or other insects. Having polluted indoor air or letting bugs eat at your home is a terrible choice to make.

Interior air pollutants are continuously emitted from air fresheners, furniture, carpets, draperies, and other fabrics. If you put stuff in your house to make it smell nice, it is emitting toxins that must be dealt with in your liver.

Have you ever had to clean the cloudy, sticky stuff off the inside of your vehicle's windshield in the middle of summer? That sticky residue consists of chemicals gassing out of the plastics used to manufacture vehicles.

Unless, of course, you are a smoker, in which case the plastic gases are combining with smoke by-products to make a very interesting mix you inhale with every breath you take while in that vehicle. Since most vehicles have a heater and air conditioner, it is uncommon to drive with the windows down to expel toxic fumes, so they stay trapped in there.

Some toxin sources may only be present periodically. Intermittent release of toxins comes from smoking materials (cigars, cigarette, or pipe smoke) or from appliances that are only functioning occasionally. Think about the stoves, heaters, and furnaces that only operate when needed. Cleaning products, glues, paints, pesticides, herbicides, or solvents like paint strippers are only used when needed, but their gases remain in the air of your buildings for a long time.

Do you open your windows to allow cross-breeze ventilation to expel indoor pollutants? Or do you keep the house closed to avoid street noise? Is it important for you to keep the heated or cooled air you have spent so much money on inside instead of letting it escape to the outside? Do the windows in your workplace open or are they sealed with a mechanical ventilation system moving the air from one room to the next, and then recirculating it?

Mechanical air moving systems do not exchange polluted air for fresh air. They only move the toxins from one area to another. Fresh air should be allowed to enter any building, but that is not the case.

Buildings are full of indoor pollutants because toxins are not being expelled. Apartment buildings may be worse than single-family homes. The sheer volume of people populating an apartment building increases the amount of toxins being produced in such a building.

With apartments, there are more building materials in the structure, more furnishings in the building, and more pesticides and cleaning chemicals being used by more families, etc. This all adds up to greater amounts of indoor pollutants being produced and staying in apartment buildings than single-family dwellings.

Irritation to the eyes, nose, or throat may accompany headaches, asthma, dizziness, or fatigue after only short exposure to toxins. It's easy to blame symptoms such as these on causes other than indoor pollution. Insidious and more serious long-term health risks may take years to appear.

Most people never consider the cause of their illness to be the unhealthy air trapped in the buildings they frequent. Some ancient societies believed air "went bad" and would make people sick. While the air does not spoil, it can be tainted with pollutants that make people ill.

It is difficult for people to believe their building is making them sick. Particularly when they suffer a serious illness. This is especially true if they have lived or worked in that building for several years.

Then there are the hypersensitivity reactions that may only appear after long-term exposure to indoor pollutants.

It is not uncommon in our day and age for people to become sensitive to chemicals. This is because of the liver becoming overloaded to where it can no longer remove toxins via the normal excretory pathways.

When your liver is overloaded because of repeated exposure to chemical toxins in buildings, it often results in an "allergic reaction" such as sneezing and watery eyes. Chemicals causing allergic reactions are often found with commonly used cleaning products.

The association between your newly gained sensitivity and chemicals may become evident when you walk through the cleaning products aisle in the supermarket. If you sneeze after entering the cleaning products aisle in the supermarket or your eyes water, you may have an overloaded liver that can no longer rid your body of chemicals efficiently. It is one sign you can monitor as you re-establish the excretory functions of your liver.

Sometimes you need to be a detective. If you immediately have allergic symptoms when you enter your home or place of business, and the symptoms lessen awhile after leaving the building, suspect an indoor pollutant as the culprit. However, you now must figure out which chemical in that environment is causing you problems. You have two options.

The first option is to begin the arduous task of sorting out which cleaning product, air freshener, etc. is the culprit. Hopefully, there is only one causing your problems. If there is more than one symptom-inducing chemical in that environment, it becomes much more difficult to isolate which ones are causing the problems.

The second option is to apply a concerted effort to detoxify your liver so toxins cease to elicit an allergic reaction. Assuming it is your overloaded liver causing the symptoms, this approach will prevent the toxins from causing your allergic reaction. Now you don't have to be a detective. It's your choice.

So how will you know if there is sufficient ventilation in your home or office to at least reduce the toxin concentration? You can look for areas that have stale air, or see if there is mold growing on books, shoes, or other items that may sit unattended for a while.

Is there excess moisture condensation on the windows or walls in the winter? This can encourage mold formation, which is a toxin. Everything seems to be a toxin that might cause you problems. It's frustrating, but there is a solution, as you shall soon see.

Air cleaners can reduce toxin concentrations in buildings by reducing particulate matter (dust) in the air before you breathe them in. Smaller air cleaning units are not as capable as larger units in performing air-cleansing functions, so you must have the correct size unit for the square footage inside your building. However, be aware that air cleaners do not reduce gas pollutants like radon, chemicals pollutants, or smoke. They only remove particles of debris from the air.

Air cleaners must move a large amount of air to be effective and must be well maintained to continue functioning at top efficiency. Reducing the number of indoor pollutants will not totally remove the problem. However, cleansing the air will minimize the amount of indoor toxins resulting in less stress on your liver. This gives your liver a better chance of keeping up with the volume of toxins it must excrete daily.

How important is it to reduce the volume of indoor pollutants? It's very important.

For example, the smoke from burning tobacco products contains a complex mixture of over four thousand compounds. Over forty of these are known cancer-causing agents. But does this really affect you, and your liver, if you do not smoke yourself but only live in a house or share an office with a smoker?

Of course it does. Approximately three thousand lung cancer deaths occur each year in non-smokers that can be contributed to smoke pollution. The Environmental Protection Agency estimates that between one hundred fifty thousand and three hundred thousand infants develop lower respiratory infections from this form of pollution. These infections are severe enough to result in about seven thousand five hundred to fifteen thousand hospitalizations per year. That's a major problem that must be addressed.

The only effective way to rid yourself of tobacco related indoor pollutants is to bar smoking from your house or work area. This is one of the easiest forms of indoor toxin sources to get rid of. Stopping the out-gassing from your carpet and furniture is tremendously more difficult.

Chapter Fourteen

Formaldehyde

What other types of items can cause indoor gas emissions?

It would take a book unto itself, and maybe an entire library, to list all the toxins and their sources. Therefore, to explore this question, we will look at formaldehyde as an example.

Organic compounds, like formaldehyde, can cause tissue-specific autoimmune reactions. Polluting compounds such as this are so common and their effects so alarming that they have developed special laboratory tests to detect them.

Formaldehyde is an important chemical used in industry to make building materials and many household products. Another common source of it is smoking or using non-vented fuel-burning appliances such as gas stoves or kerosene space heaters inside a building.

Formaldehyde is found in common items such as clothing, draperies, glues, adhesives, paints, and other coating products. When it emanates from materials found in households, it can be a major source of indoor pollution and is often found in strong concentrations.

The single most important source of formaldehyde toxins comes from pressed wood products that are made with adhesives containing urea-formaldehyde resin. You will find this type of pressed wood product in sub-flooring, shelves, furniture, kitchen cabinets, and wall paneling.

The emission of formaldehyde is so prevalent and worrisome that the Department of Housing and Urban Development (HUD) only permits the use of plywood or particleboard in mobile home construction that is specially formulated to limit formaldehyde emissions.

Prefabricated homes were targeted because of the large amount of pressed wood products used in their construction and their small size. Unsurprisingly, mobile homes have very high concentrations of formaldehyde inside, which is a concern.

Formaldehyde emissions reduce with time resulting in lesser concentrations as years pass by. That's OK if you don't breathe for a few years otherwise your poor, over-worked liver must transform the formaldehyde into a form that can be excreted.

Using formaldehyde as an example of indoor toxins gives you a good idea of how common items within your home can contribute to indoor pollution. Pollution such as this affects your liver and may contribute to you having an unhealthy accumulation of body fat.

Chapter Fifteen

How Toxins Sneak Into Your Home

To further explore how toxins sneak into people's homes and businesses we will single out pesticides. For the sake of discussion, you can assume other poisons such as herbicides may be viewed similarly.

They estimated that seventy-five percent of American households have used at least one pesticide indoors within the last year. When toxins are found indoors, they appear in strong concentrations. This is worrisome because measurable levels of up to a dozen pesticides can be found in homes.

Here's an interesting fact. The quantity of pesticides found in homes appears to be greater than can be explained by recent pesticide use in those homes.

WOW! This stuff multiplies!

Well, not really.

It is suspected that contaminated soil or dust finds its way into your house when the windows and doors are opened or is tracked into the house on your shoes. Don't forget about the pesticides that are stored in your house or settled on flat surfaces. They're still releasing fumes and toxins into the air as they sit there. These sources of pesticide fumes add up to a lot of airborne pesticide toxins over time that are not related to any current pest problem existing in your house.

Pesticides are troublesome to your inability to lose weight because they are usually xenoestrogens. That is, hormones that mimic the effects of estrogen.

Remember the prevalence of pesticides when you are reading about the effects of estrogen on fat creation and retention in a later chapter. That discussion will drive home the importance of the presence of pesticides in your environment and their effect on your waistline.

Pesticides encompass many chemicals that are used for an array of pests. Those for insects are called insecticides while termiticides are for termites. Rodenticides are for rodents like mice and rats. Then there are the pesticides that are not usually thought of as pesticides. These are the fungicides for fungus and disinfectants for germs.

Pesticides can be applied by several methods. They come in powders, liquid sprays, liquid form to be poured, sticks, crystals, aerosols, and even "balls" such as mothballs.

Any word that ends with "-cide" means it is used to kill. It will kill little bugs and it will kill you if the concentrations are high enough.

To put some light on the extent of pesticide use, it may be useful to know that way back in 1990, the American Association of Poison Control Centers reported that approximately 79,000 children were poisoned with household pesticides and required medical care. So, this is not a new problem and has been going on for a long time. You must ask how high those figures are today with more children and an increasing number of pesticides showing up in our homes. In 2008, pesticides were the ninth most common substance reported to poison control centers. That's rather disturbing.

Believe it or not, fungicides are commonly found in consumable products. Food processors spray fungicides on grain while in storage to discourage the formation of fungus, which would ruin the grain. Yes, the FDA allows a certain level of fungicides and other harmful "stuff" into your food and water, but it always states it as being "permissible" levels. Please understand that your body may not agree with the FDA's assessment of the situation.

Those permissible levels are based on the amount that will kill you or cause immediate and recognizable harm. It does not consider whether long-term exposure will overload your liver or if repeated contact over time will result in an unhealthy accumulation of toxins within your body. This is an important distinction to make when discussing the effects of toxins on your body.

Ditto for rodenticides as mice and rats are drawn to grain storage areas. Rodenticides may therefore be found in minute amounts in your food.

Rodenticides are usually found in very low levels that will not cause disease. However, your liver must still work to expel these toxins from your body regardless of how small the amount.

One form of pesticide, the cyclodiene pesticides, has caught the attention of the Environmental Protection Agency. Cyclodienes have been shown to cause long-term damage to the liver, affect the central nervous system, and increase the incidence of cancer.

Let's pay attention to the liver damage right now. Why do you think the liver is damaged by cyclodiene?

Is it because the liver concentrates poisons so they can be excreted? What if the liver is not working correctly? What does the liver do when concentrations are getting higher and higher, and it can't get rid of this stuff?

My, My. That's what this book is about, isn't it? Can you see how a single chemical compound can affect your liver? What about the thousands of other compounds you are exposed to every day? The situation quickly becomes mind numbing.

How much do environmental toxins truly affect you? To find out, a comprehensive study was performed and concluded environmental toxins play a much larger role in cancer development than was previously thought.

In that study, over 44,000 pairs of twins were assessed for potential connections that may lead to cancer. It might be assumed there would be a huge correlation between health and disease among twins. Wouldn't you think?

The inherited factors that led to breast cancer (breast cancer was the disease being studied) were estimated at only thirty percent. Due to this finding, researchers concluded that inherited genetic factors made only a small contribution to breast cancer onset. The principal cause of cancer was deemed, at least by these researchers, to be environmentally related.

Many fat-soluble chemicals are stored in body fat. That's why you are warned not to eat fatty fish like salmon, particularly those from the Great Lakes, more than once a week, and not at all if you are a small child or pregnant. The fat-soluble chemicals have accumulated in the fish's fat and that concentrated mix gets transferred straight into you when you eat the fish. Talk about the ultimate payback. Sheesh!

OK, so now you know toxins are all around you most of your daily lives. However, environmental toxins may only be one of many sources of toxins. The largest contributor of toxins overloading your liver may come from your own body and this situation must be corrected if you want to have any hope of having a liver that can detoxify everything it must.

Oh Brother! What now?

Well, let's get to it and look at the Leaky Gut Syndrome.

Chapter Sixteen

Leaky Gut Syndrome

Uh-Oh. This sounds bad.

It is.

Unfortunately, it is also very common.

Leaky Gut Syndrome is also known as "Intestinal Permeability." We will use the term Leaky Gut Syndrome because it is more graphic and will better help you understand what is going on. Also, if you research this condition on the Internet, some articles you find may call it Intestinal Permeability instead of Leaky Gut Syndrome. Now that you know both names it goes by you will not be confused.

In simple terms, Leaky Gut Syndrome is a condition in which the intestines, or gut, "leak" everything from partially digested food to bacteria into the bloodstream. The importance of a leaking gut is that you should remedy it prior to trying to fix the ability of your liver to detoxify your body.

What causes a leaky gut? Leaky gut is caused by toxic pesticide residue (from the environment or your foods), refined sugar, refined carbohydrates, bacteria, and from nutritional deficiencies that either allow the gut to degrade or which do not allow proper gut functioning to occur. There are other causes, and we will address them shortly because it is important for you to understand how this all works. That way you can formulate a plan to get yourself back on track and lose some weight.

Anti-inflammatory drugs such as aspirin, ibuprofen, and many others can contribute to a leaky gut. Many ill-informed people eat medications like candy and this habit has long-term detrimental effects.

Leaky Gut Syndrome affects the lining of the intestines. The gastro-intestinal tract, or gut, performs several functions such as digesting food to break it down into small usable components. Then the gut absorbs the digested food so it can cross into the bloodstream. Nutrients like vitamins and minerals are taken into the bloodstream via protein carriers that "grab" the nutrients and pull them across the gut wall to be dumped into the blood. Vitamins and minerals are then carried by the blood to distant reaches of the body where they are needed.

The gastro-intestinal tract contains a major part of the body's chemical detoxification system and contains antibodies and immunoglobulins that will defend against infection entering your body through your digestive system. It is your first line of defense in that area of your body, so a healthy, non-leaking gut is very important to your overall health and to your waistline.

Let's look at the act of digestion for a moment. It's not too difficult to understand what is occurring, and it's very interesting since all this stuff is going on in your belly without you having to think about it.

Potassium, magnesium, chloride, sodium, and free fatty acids just diffuse through the cells of the gut. In layperson's terms, this means these nutrients drift through the cells to get into the bloodstream. This is normal.

The active transport method absorbs nutrients like amino acids, fatty acids, vitamins, minerals, and glucose (blood sugar). This is where the proteins mentioned above "grab" the nutrients and pull them across the gut wall to dump them into the bloodstream.

There is a third way that substances pass through the gut wall to get into the bloodstream. This third route involves desmosomes.

Desmosomes are spaces between the cells of the gut that are normally sealed. However, when the intestine lining gets inflamed and irritated, these spaces open a bit. This allows molecules that would normally be too large to traverse the gut wall to sneak through it on their way into the bloodstream.

As the intestinal lining becomes more inflamed, it allows larger and larger molecules to escape across the gut wall and into the bloodstream. Undigested food particles, toxins, disease-producing bacteria, viruses, and everything else that's in the gut passes straight into the bloodstream. This is where problems occur.

Most of the items crossing the gut wall are made of protein. Protein triggers a reaction from the immune system of the body. The immune system immediately forms antibodies to those proteins because they are not normally found in the blood and are therefore targeted as being "foreign invaders" to the body.

The action of the antibodies causes the production of oxidants. Oxidants cause all types of irritation and inflammation throughout the entire body, starting problems far removed from the gut itself. You may have heard of antioxidants that battle against these oxidants and the damage they cause inside your body.

The resulting symptoms from the presence of oxidants may include things like belly pain, joint pain, confusion, fatigue, abnormal amounts of abdominal gas, indigestion, "fuzzy" or "foggy" thinking, nervousness, mood swings, aggressive behavior, and/or poor immune responses that may cause frequent bouts of cold and flu-like symptoms and other illnesses.

Leaky Gut Syndrome has been associated with a diverse list of symptoms, including but not limited to:

• Recurrent bladder or vaginal infections.

• Poor memory.

• Frequent diarrhea or constipation (go figure!).

• Skin rashes.

• Anxiety.

• Irritable bowel syndrome, Celiac Disease, and even Crohn's Disease.

• Food allergies and sensitivities.

• Eczema and Psoriasis.

•Hives.

•Acne.

•Allergies.

• Inflamed joints and arthritis.

• Chronic Fatigue Syndrome.

• Liver dysfunction (This one is a large part of what we are discussing in this book.)

• Autoimmune diseases such as rheumatoid arthritis and lupus erythematosus.

In many autoimmune diseases such as rheumatoid arthritis, they have reported encouraging results when people suffering from this affliction address their food allergies via dietary changes. Digestive enzymes also help by breaking down foods, especially those foods the arthritis sufferers are allergic to, and by healing the leaking gut to stop the flow of allergens from the intestines.

Recent research supports the theory that wheat and dairy allergies cause many autoimmune system disorders. There appear to be segments of protein found in wheat gluten and dairy products that mimic protein normally found in the body.

While the research is ongoing and far from being conclusive, wheat gluten protein may be molecularly similar to a glycocollagen protein found in joint cartilage. When anti-bodies form to combat the foreign proteins of wheat gluten that leaked across the gut barrier, they cannot discern between wheat gluten proteins and glycocollagen proteins in the joints, so they attack both. The result is rheumatoid arthritis.

They have shown that up to two percent of protein can avoid being digested. These proteins are absorbed and end up in the bloodstream as intact allergens. That leads to many problems.

The leaky gut can also lead to environmental illnesses.

Environmental illness? Do you mean having a sneezing fit every time you walk down the cleaning products aisle in the supermarket might mean you have a leaky gut?

Yep. It is possibly a sign of an overloaded liver, as we have already discussed. That makes sense since the leaky gut is a major, and maybe the number one contributor, to the formation of an overloaded liver. Are you seeing how the leaky gut and overloaded liver are related? It's never just one item that causes your body to malfunction. Everything is interrelated, and problems are usually multi-faceted.

What that means to you is there will never be a cure-all for all your problems. You must be diligent, work through each problem, and then move onto the next one. Life is difficult, but it is survivable if you know what to do and then do it.

So, what are some of the other causes of Leaky Gut Syndrome that may be negatively affecting you and your health?

Naturally, stress is involved. Stress is always involved, so just get it out of your life right now, OK? Yeah, right! If it were only that easy…

That's the problem with the conditions we are discussing. Everyday occurrences and items that are part of your normal life and habits cause them. Because of this, we will take a systematic approach, one that will allow you to improve your health without having to move to undeveloped and less polluted parts of the world.

Reality is reality. You must work within the constraints of what you are willing to do to improve your health. Otherwise, you will ignore everything and continue down the path to ill health for what will be the rest of your shortened and illness-ridden life.

Intestinal infections can cause a leaky gut because they directly damage the gut wall. Candida infection is common these days because of the antibiotics consumed for many ailments. Antibiotics not only kill the bacteria causing illness, but they also wipe out the "good" bacteria that act as the first line of defense against "bad" bacteria and yeast infections such as Candida albicans.

When the good bacteria (also known as the beneficial bacteria) are present, they occupy space in your gut. Literally, there is no room for the bad bacteria and/or yeast to get a foothold to grow upon. Using antibiotics can kill all the good bacteria, which makes space for the bad bacteria and/or yeast to move in. The fertile ground of your gut is inviting unwanted bacteria and/or yeast to set up housekeeping and by removing the good bacteria, it opens the floodgates to bad infestations.

Years ago, my dog had an ear infection, and the veterinarian prescribed antibiotics for her. He also gave us a syringe full of "good" doggie gut bacteria. The vet instructed me to squirt half of the beneficial bacteria down her throat upon arriving home and administer the other half two weeks later, after the antibiotic regimen was complete. That makes perfect sense to me. What makes little sense is why they give good bacteria to dogs after antibiotic therapy but not to humans? Pets may get better health care than the humans caring for them!

Has your medical doctor ever given you good bacteria along with your antibiotic prescription? I doubt it. If they have, stay with that doctor because they know what they are doing.

After taking a course of antibiotics, eating yogurt or buttermilk with active cultures can help reintroduce good gut bacteria to your system, but these foods are not as good as having the natural bacterial levels that should be there. Products containing good bacteria are available at well-stocked pharmacies and do not require a prescription.

These products should be refrigerated both in the store and at home until consumed. Ask the pharmacist for them. Inquire about products containing Lactobacillus bifidus, acidophilus, or L. casei, and they'll guide you in the right direction. These organisms will help restore colonization by normal gut bacteria.

Why doctors do not tell their patients about the "bacteria paradox" every time they prescribe antibiotics may be a sign they are not familiar with this problem. More doctors must learn how to work with the body instead of against it. Pills are not always the answer to your problems. It is good practice to understand the mechanisms going on within your body and then create a situation so it can heal itself.

Environmental contaminants, excessive alcohol consumption, certain medications (including many over-the-counter medications), and a poor diet can also cause Leaky Gut Syndrome. Most Americans may be susceptible to Leaky Gut Syndrome from their eating habits alone.

But isn't the job of the gut wall to move nutrients across to the bloodstream? So, isn't a leaky gut a good thing? Doesn't it just speed up this process? No, it's not a good thing.

Remember discussing active transport where a protein "grabs" a mineral or vitamin then pulls it across the gut wall? Well, those proteins are damaged and can't do their job. The result is a person with a leaky gut who is susceptible to vitamin and mineral deficiency. That's not a good thing. Many vital functions of your body depend on vitamins and minerals for normal functioning.

If mineral deficiency occurs, all kinds of symptoms may result. For instance, magnesium deficiency can elicit muscle spasms. Copper deficiency may cause high cholesterol. The real kicker is that you will never know what is causing these strange symptoms to occur because you are unaware of the true cause of your afflictions.

With a leaky gut comes the flow of foreign proteins into the bloodstream. Remember that the body responds to foreign proteins by forming antibodies to them? Well, these antibodies also attack the joints and other connective tissues, potentially resulting in conditions such as fibromyalgia, lupus, multiple sclerosis, and rheumatoid arthritis.

The popular press has recently recognized Leaky Gut Syndrome and is reporting on a plethora of diseases including asthma and arthritis that are resulting from this condition. It's good to see the popular press recognize this common ailment, though we're still not hearing enough about this pervasive and devastating condition.

Chapter Seventeen

What Should You Do?

So, what are you going to do? Not eat anything? Hide in your basement and tremble in fear?

Well, you can grow your own food, which is a great thing to do if you have the time and inclination. But for most of us the most practical option is to keep your liver healthy and capable of excreting toxins as soon as possible from your body.

Oh, and make sure you take a food supplement supplying glutamine. They found glutamine helps maintain the gut wall so viruses, bacteria, and food antigens cannot invade the body. It is the main nutritional factor helping to maintain and repair the gut lining, which sloughs off every three days. That's a lot of continual maintenance and repair of your gut requiring the daily consumption of essential nutrition needed to maintain your body when cells need to be repaired or replaced.

Digestive enzymes are helpful because they aid in digesting foods more completely, breaking foods down into their constituent parts so whole proteins are no longer present. When enzymes "tear apart" these proteins, they prevent them from leaking across the gut wall intact and disorienting your immune system. Pancreatic digestive enzymes include proteases to digest proteins, amylases for digesting starches, and lipases which digest fats. Using pepsin along with the enzymes listed above can be helpful for conditions such as diabetes where the pancreas is not operating at its optimal levels.

One example of how digestive enzymes can be beneficial to us is illustrated by a study that explored the use of Papain, a derivative of papaya. Papain was observed "to be effective in celiac disease patients by digesting the wheat gluten and rendering it harmless" according to the authors of the study. That's a good thing to know as celiac disease is a hard condition to manage, and many prepared foods have wheat products "hidden" in them, making avoiding wheat products difficult. However, if you suffer from celiac disease or leaky gut, you may want to investigate the use of papain or anything else that is supposed to help these types of conditions with great caution.

It takes quite a while to heal the gut. Be patient. Some healthcare practitioners feel it takes a minimum of three months to heal the gut. That's why you will need to adopt a healthier lifestyle to aid the repair process.

Having a healthy gut will help your liver function better, which helps in the achievement of a healthier body weight.

That's why all your previous weight loss diets failed. You didn't have enough information to see the big picture, and what information you had could have been misleading or misguided. Therefore, you were doomed to fail from the start in your quest for a healthier body weight.

With those weight loss diets, you weren't given all the information you needed to understand why you must weave healthier living habits, a healthy gut, and a liver with improved function into your current lifestyle. Knowledge is power, and you must have the correct knowledge to achieve your goals.

Unfortunately, Leaky Gut Syndrome appears to be on the rise. This is not surprising, as the sheer number of environmental and dietary factors you encounter daily are working against you. Beware the "quick cure" as some of these "wonder cures" are detrimental to the healing process. For example, you often see aloe vera suggested as a soothing elixir to the gut tube. In reality, this bitter herb, when taken as a concentrated liquid, can irritate an already inflamed intestinal tract. Be careful.

So, what can you do if you suspect you have a leaky gut? Well, you can just clean up your act and follow the proper nutritional guidelines to heal your gut, or you can be tested. Seeing a Functional Medicine Doctor or other healthcare professional well versed in nutritional therapies is strongly recommended so they can guide you in treating your leaking gut. Testing for a leaky gut has its benefits because you can retest later to verify the problem has been corrected.

A good book to read for more information about functional medicine is *The Disease Delusion: Conquering the Causes of Chronic Illness for a Healthier, Longer, and Happier Life* by Dr. Jeffrey S. Bland. This is a fascinating field of study and one you should know more about. If you are interested, I put a link to Dr. Bland's book on my website at www.DEHeil.com to make it convenient for you and to make sure you get the correct one.

The standard test for Leaky Gut Syndrome is the mannitol and lactulose test. Mannitol and lactulose are water-soluble molecules that are not used by the body. Since the body does not use them, every bit that is absorbed is excreted. The absorption of these compounds can be accurately and easily measured since the body excretes them in the urine.

A healthy gut absorbs mannitol while it only absorbs lactulose in minute quantities. The test involves drinking a solution containing both substances. Urine is collected for six hours and the amount of these substances in the urine reflects how much was absorbed. Pretty easy, isn't it?

A healthy gut will show high levels of mannitol being absorbed and only a scant amount of lactulose being absorbed. A leaky gut will allow large amounts of both substances to be absorbed.

If low levels of each are found in the urine, then there is a general malabsorption of all nutrients. That situation can lead to nutritional deficiencies even though you are eating a healthy diet. In this case, further investigation is warranted to determine why necessary nutrients are not being absorbed. Follow your doctor's instructions. They will guide you through this.

The results from the first mannitol/lactulose test can be used to make comparisons with later tests after you take corrective action. This allows you to monitor whether your interventions are making a difference with your leaky gut problem or not. That's much preferable to just guessing if your gut is functioning correctly or not.

If Leaky Gut Syndrome is a major component of your problem, you will need some help in getting it under control. That's why it's important to form a good relationship with a healthcare professional who understands proper nutrition and its effects on your body. Their input will guide you through a systematic program to address all these problems in an organized and logical manner. Their education and experience will be invaluable to you.

So how does a dysfunctional liver cause an unhealthy accumulation of fat in your body? To illustrate what is taking place, let's look at a single situation, such as that occurring with estrogen, to better understand what is taking place.

Estrogen-like substances in the environment affect everyone. Let's take a hard look at this cantankerous little hormone that may cause you such grief.

Chapter Eighteen

Estrogen and Fat Production

UH-OH! Hormones.

Estrogen!! Double UH-OH!

Estrogen is primarily thought to be a female hormone and, because men are not sure what it does, the mere mentioning of it strikes fear into their hearts. Yep, men seem to associate estrogen with women and PMS. Most men have learned to fear estrogen and anything else associated with "that time of the month."

Of course, estrogen is much more involved in human physiology and is not only a female hormone that "does something to women." The belief that estrogen is only found in women is simply the erroneous thinking of shell-shocked men!

Estrogen affects men too.

All your body's hormones, whether they are considered masculine or feminine, are present in everyone to differing degrees. If one hormone is high in concentration, one effect will be produced. If another is low in concentration, you get another effect. And while it may come as a surprise, both estrogen and testosterone, the presumed "masculine" hormone, are present to varying degrees in both men and women.

Hormones levels are constantly being adjusted by competition amongst hormones in a very intricate system of balance and counterbalance. So begins our discussion of excessive estrogen in our bodies.

Why should we even be discussing estrogen? Because increased estrogen suppresses fat burning. Remember when we discussed body fat and what causes it to be deposited where you don't want it to be and in greater amounts than you're comfortable with? One reason women have higher concentrations of body fat is that estrogen encourages their bodies to store fat. Considering we are interested in losing fat and keeping it off, this seems like an important topic worth discussing. Right?

We will discuss the aspects of estrogen pertaining to fat burning, fat retention, and how increases in estrogen levels occur in the body.

Chapter Nineteen

Estrogen Dominance

A much more detailed and extensive discussion of hormones, particularly estrogen and progesterone, another hormone typically associated with female physiology, can be found in the book entitled *What Your Doctor May Not Tell You About Premenopause* by John R. Lee, M.D., Jesse Hanley, M.D., and Virginia Hopkins. For those readers seeking additional material regarding hormonal fluctuations, this book comes highly recommended. It is written for the layperson, so it is very understandable and easy to read.

Dr. Lee speaks of a state called "estrogen dominance" where the amount of estrogen is much greater than the amount of progesterone in your body. Estrogen dominance can be problematic as the role of progesterone is to balance the effects of estrogen. When the natural ratio of estrogen to progesterone is skewed, unwanted side effects occur.

Estrogen dominance is important to our discussion of healthy amounts of body fat because it has been linked to an increase in fat around the belly, hips, and thighs. Do I have your attention now? Good. There are more juicy tidbits coming up, so pay close attention.

Estrogen dominance also causes sluggish metabolism and thyroid dysfunction, which mimics a hypothyroid condition. Both situations work against your attempts to achieve a lower amount of body fat.

Estrogen dominance has several medical and dietary causes. Interestingly, people create most of these situations themselves. This means you have near total control over whether estrogen dominance affects you.

Many women take birth control pills, which increases the amount of estrogen available to their bodies. More germane to our discussion is excessive caloric intake (also known as overeating!) that is the standard in American eating habits these days and increases the chance of estrogen dominance developing. The scarcity of consuming fresh fruits and vegetables, combined with the popularity of sugars and refined starches in the average American diet, can lead to estrogen dominance.

Uh-oh. That's a lot of dietary causes relating to estrogen dominance. Fortunately, this is a book about correcting your eating habits.

A leading factor in the estrogen dominance scenario is a liver with impaired functioning. A healthy, fully functioning liver can break down excess estrogen while an overloaded liver cannot regulate excess estrogen. Are you seeing the causal relationship between estrogen dominance, unhealthy amounts of body fat, and a sluggish liver?

Medical therapies for endometriosis, a condition maintained by high levels of estrogen, try to lower estrogen levels by suppressing estrogen production. An alternative to this pharmaceutical solution is to strengthen your liver so it can more efficiently break down and remove excess estrogen from your bloodstream.

The liver regulates estrogen by breaking it down through oxidation and conjugation. Mostly, conjugated estrogen is excreted in the bile, with a small amount excreted in the urine. Because estrogen dominance accompanies certain types of liver disorders it helps confirm the important role of the liver in estrogen breakdown and excretion.

One research paper describes the process by which estrogen breakdown goes awry because of inefficient liver performance. When that occurs, it results in the formation of a cancer-causing metabolite. Staving off cancer is at least as important as losing weight, isn't it?

The good news is that a proper diet containing the correct essential fatty acids such as omega-3 fatty acids and fresh vegetables like broccoli, cauliflower, onions, and beans stops the manufacture of this cancer-causing metabolite.

***

Estrogen and Cancer

Let's take a minute and discuss the carcinogenic (cancer causing) aspects of estrogen. Understanding the relationship between estrogen and cancer must be at least as important as its relationship to making fat, right? By recognizing the relationship between how estrogen is metabolized, broken down, excreted, and the relationships these biological processes have with cancer, you can better appreciate how important diet is to the entire system and your weight loss efforts.

Most people think of estrogen as a single compound, but it's not. It is several distinct substances your body naturally produces.

Why talk about cancer in a book that helps you lower body fat? It's because the studies dealing with cancer have been a watershed of new information we can use to illustrate how the liver interacts with hormones like estrogen. As we progress through this book, you will better understand the effects of estrogen, why the liver is an important part of this scenario, and its direct effects on body fat.

Most laboratory researchers and oncologists agree that a combination of factors like behavioral, dietary, genetic, and hormonal components are implicated in the formation of conditions such as breast cancer.

It is known that breast cancer risk increases with an early onset of the first menstrual period, late onset of menopause (both of which increase the time estrogen is actively produced and circulating in the body), long-term use of estrogen-based oral contraceptives, and administering estrogen replacement therapies (also known as "hormone replacement therapy" which is more commonly called "HRT"). Elevated estrogen levels and uncommonly long-term exposure to estrogen may also factor into a perpetually unhealthy accumulation of body fat.

Estrogen is broken down, or detoxified, into several metabolites that are then excreted from the body. Of course, that depends on whether everything works as it should. The two main metabolites of interest to this discussion are known as 2-hydroxyesterone and 16-hydroxyesterone (just remember #2 and #16).

Now, follow me on this. It is important to understand what is going on here early in our discussion because it is directly related to everything we will talk about concerning fat burning.

To keep it simple, 2-hydroxyesterone is good and 16-hydroxyesterone is bad.

The chemical pathway the liver takes to form 2-hydroxyesterone is called the C-2 pathway. Following this intuitive line of labeling, the chemical pathway the liver takes to form 16-hydroxyesterone is called the C-16 pathway. That is simple enough so far, right?

To reduce the incidence of cancer formation, it is better to shuttle as much estrogen down the C-2 pathway to be broken down and excreted. The C-2 pathway makes estrogen metabolites that pose less of a cancerous risk to your body, while the C-16 pathway manufactures estrogen metabolites that nurture malignant cancer formation.

Eating fresh fruits, raw vegetables, and whole grains (particularly flaxseed) increases the amount of estrogen metabolized via the preferred C-2 pathway.

To put this into perspective and recap it all, when estrogen breaks down via the preferred C-2 pathway, it makes more of the 2-hydroxyesterone, which is less cancer causing than 16-hydroxyesterone. What you do not want happening is estrogen breaking down via the detrimental C-16 pathway because it produces more of the harmful 16-hydroxyesterone.

C-2 is good, while C-16 is bad. That's simple enough to follow, right?

So, what determines if estrogen is broken down via the preferred C-2 or the dreaded C-16 pathways? The answer is your genetic make-up and your environment (both of which you have only limited control over) and your diet and lifestyle (both of which you have total control over).

Studies have shown that women who metabolize more of their excess estrogen down the C-16 pathway, and less down the C-2 pathway, have a greater incidence of breast cancer. Again, scientists figure this is because C-16 metabolites are more prone to start cancerous activity.

One study, which followed 10,786 women over a five-and-a-half-year period, found that those developing breast cancer had much less 2-hydroxyesterone and more 16-hydroxyesterone metabolites. In this study, the women with increased 2-hydroxyesterone levels showed a forty percent decrease in the occurrence of breast cancer. That's significant.

From these studies, it appears that any variable favoring C-2 pathway metabolism over C-16 metabolism would help reduce the risk of developing breast cancer. This means any medical or dietary changes encouraging estrogen breakdown via C-2 are in your best interest. The good news is that scientists may have identified these factors. Let's explore and see what the researchers have discovered.

Estrogen is broken down using the same enzymes the liver uses to detoxify the blood. These enzymes determine whether estrogen is metabolized via the C-2 pathway or one of the other less desirable pathways, such as the C-16 pathway. These enzymes direct metabolic "traffic," telling the excess estrogen where to go.

If the C-2 pathway can be coaxed into shouldering most of the estrogen metabolism, while C-16 pathway use is lessened, cancer risks can be reduced. Neat, huh?

Now, let's inspect what can coax the beneficial C-2 pathway to do most of this job.

Chapter Twenty

Phytonutrients to the Rescue

So, how do you make your liver shuttle estrogen down the C-2 pathway instead of down the C-16 pathway? The answer is that you change your diet to include more fresh fruits and raw vegetables, consuming the same food items used to reduce fat retention. It's those important enzymes and phytonutrients to the rescue once again!

If you can reduce your chance of getting cancer and improve your liver function by eating the same foods, why wouldn't you do it? It is a smart thing to do, but it is up to you.

But what types of fruits and vegetables best supply the needed enzymes to the liver so the C-2 pathway is favored? Well, the Brassica family of vegetables is a good place to start. These include the vegetables broccoli, Brussels sprouts, cauliflower, kale, kohlrabi, rutabaga, mustard, turnip, and Bok choy.

Other foods such as flaxseed and whole grains have a large effect on shuttling estrogen down the C-2 pathway instead of down the C-16 pathway. These recommended foods contain the phytonutrients involved in influencing estrogen production and metabolism.

Lignans, the source of these phytonutrients in grains and flaxseed, have proved effective in inhibiting the spread of breast cancer cells when tested in cell cultures, so eating these foods makes sense.

While cell cultures are not directly related to living breast tissue in the body, it may be helpful to eat more lignan-rich grains and flaxseed just to be on the safe side until more testing can be done. It won't hurt you and has many other beneficial effects.

Why wait for a dangerous situation to appear if you can take simple, inexpensive steps toward preventing it in the first place? This the idea behind preventative medicine, isn't it? Getting with the program now will help you stay healthy and be slimmer.

Things other than fresh fruits and vegetables that may affect which estrogen-metabolizing pathway is used include foods such as soy protein.

Soy protein has a plethora of nutritional components in it but the most likely candidates in reducing the threat of breast cancer are called isoflavones. The isoflavones found in soy protein cause more estrogen to be metabolized through the more beneficial C-2 pathway.

Besides soy protein, there is an isoflavone found in kudzu, a wild plant that is taking over large portions of the southern United States. Though regarded as an invasive species, kudzu is edible and has some health benefits. The good news is that the isoflavones found in kudzu also favor the C-2 estrogen metabolic pathway in a manner similar to the isoflavones in soy protein.

This is a great boon for residents of the South where kudzu is taking over. Finally, there's a good reason for folks to harvest kudzu. And because it spreads rapidly, it is readily and abundantly available.

You'll soon see what all this information has to do with an unhealthy accumulation of body fat. It's important to face the reality of the situation so you can avoid bad things from happening. And it's easy to do, it really is.

Estrogen dominance is a biological reality in our society. Men, women, children, and animals are all susceptible to suffering from the effects of estrogen dominance. That's because we find the chief causes of it in our environment. The pollutants we discussed before can cause excessive estrogen production or an overabundant manufacture of chemical compounds that mimic the effects of estrogen. Both situations will give you the same unwanted effect.

Plastics, pesticides, herbicides, auto exhaust emissions, hormones in the meat you eat, the cosmetic products you apply to your skin, and even the out-gassing of chemicals from your home furnishings can increase the level of estrogen in your body. The effects of these extra hormones will take a negative toll on your body, while you're ignorant of what's causing the problems.

Headaches, sinus problems, asthma, dry eyes, or chilly hands and feet may be signs of estrogen dominance. These are symptoms I hear about every day from patients suffering from estrogen dominance. These types of symptoms are so common they are being accepted as the new normal. They are not normal so do not fall into that mental trap.

Everyone seems to have "allergies" that have their sinuses flared up. Women are always "cold" with icy hands and feet being an accepted fact of life. These are unnatural states that can, and should, be corrected.

The most common effect of estrogen dominance in women is the lack of ovulation.

Some women know when they are ovulating, and some don't. Ovulation controls when progesterone, the hormone that counterbalances estrogen, is secreted. While the menstruation cycle may appear normal, if ovulation has not occurred, the affected women may experience symptoms of Pre-Menstrual Syndrome (PMS).

PMS symptoms include mood swings, cramps, tender breasts, and even weight gain. PMS, icy hands and feet, headaches, and allergy or asthma-like symptoms are rampant these days. It didn't use to be like that, but it is now.

Soon you will see what an enormous problem this is for us today. The prevalence of estrogen (often consumed as birth control pills), or estrogen-like substances (from plastics and cosmetics) that mimic the effects of estrogen, bombard us every minute of every day.

Add to this the deficiencies in the typical American diet that reduces your body's ability to dispose of these extra estrogen-like compounds and it all makes sense.

Chapter Twenty-One

Stress and Fat Production

Then there's stress. Stress is a nebulous term we all use and recognize, but do not have a clue what it is. We say we are "under stress" or "stressed out" when we are on the verge of a nervous breakdown, but we do not recognize its effects in our everyday lives.

Stress, whether mental or physical, occurs when your body must react to an extreme situation. This involves the dumping of adrenaline (epinephrine, norepinephrine, and such) into your bloodstream, a response that triggers your "flight or fight" mechanism.

When you are scared or excited, the "flight or fight" mechanism kicks in so you can respond almost instinctively to a perceived threat. For example, when a bear surprises you in the woods, you need extra strength and endurance to either "fight" the threat or run (take "flight") and evade the threat.

That's nice. But most of us aren't confronted with bears every day… or anything even close to it. However, many of us experience a blaring alarm clock first thing in the morning. Think about this for a moment.

There you are, sleeping soundly, dreaming of warm, sandy beaches as you lounge in secure slumber. Suddenly, there is a screaming alarm clock going off a few feet from your ears. You have no clue what is happening. You awaken in a panic, ready to "fight" or "take flight" to an as-yet-unidentified threat.

Congratulations, you have just experienced your first stress of the day. Sounds silly, doesn't it? Such an everyday occurrence as the alarm clock going off can trigger stress, and you never even knew it. That's the way the body works, which is why stressors are difficult to recognize.

Moving through your morning, you experience many more stressful situations. Pretend you are late leaving your house, so you become panicked to get to work on time, which involves more dumping of adrenaline. Then you fight to get on the highway, where you know all those crazy drivers are out to kill you, right? And another adrenaline dump occurs (or maybe three or four, depending on how harrowing that has been).

Before you even get to work or otherwise begin your day, you experience many "stressful" situations, to the detriment of your body's homeostatic tranquility.

There is nothing wrong with the flight-or-fight mechanism. It's there for a very important reason. It acts as an instinctive response designed to protect us. However, when it is overused, it provokes undesirable changes in your body chemistry. One of those adverse changes is that it creates a vicious cycle perpetuating the occurrence of estrogen dominance.

According to Lee, Hanley, and Hopkins, stress increases the levels of cortisol in your bloodstream. Because cortisol and progesterone (the hormone that balances out estrogen) compete for the same receptor sites on the cells of the body, additional cortisol reduces the ability of progesterone to balance out the effects of estrogen. This leads to estrogen dominance.

Cortisol also forces glucose (blood sugar) into the body's cells, which results in a decrease in the amount of glucose in the bloodstream. The reduction of blood glucose levels commonly produces the sensation of hunger.

When you become stressed, your blood sugar drops. When your blood sugar drops, you want to eat. Why do you want to eat? Because you need to consume calories to replace the "depleted" blood sugar reserves your body thinks it's missing. So, you snack. As is usually the case, you end up eating the wrong foods, foods that supply a fast infusion of sugar into your bloodstream while offering little nutritional value to the rest of your body.

The resulting fluctuation of blood sugar levels from sugary foods (or foods that are converted to sugar like bananas, grains, etc.) leads to the release of adrenaline and cortisol, which depletes the adrenal glands, tiring them out.

A visual representation of such a cycle would look something like this:

Stress leads to increased cortisol, which leads to estrogen dominance. Increased estrogen dominance leads to increased eating and increased fat storage. That leads to more estrogen dominance causing anxiety and increased adrenaline which depletes your adrenal glands. Depleted adrenal glands cause still more estrogen dominance which repeats the cycle over and over again becoming a self-perpetuating cycle of stress, eating, and increased fat deposits.

Other factors can exacerbate this vicious cycle, such as caffeine. Did you ever wonder why the caffeine in soda, coffee or tea causes you to feel more awake and energetic? The answer is that caffeine makes the adrenal glands excrete more adrenaline than they would under normal circumstances.

The artificial dumping of adrenaline caused by caffeine consumption overworks the adrenal glands and they become fatigued. Depleted adrenal glands put you right into the vicious cycle that leads to estrogen dominance, and estrogen dominance leads to fat retention. That's what you do not want.

A lack of sufficient nutrients in your diet adds to the early fatiguing of the adrenal glands by denying them the nutritional building blocks they need to replenish and repair themselves. Just as overworked muscles need time to recover after strenuous activity, so do the adrenal glands. We should minimize unnecessary stressing of the adrenal glands by avoiding stress and caffeine as much as possible.

A lack of nutrients, especially a lack of dietary enzymes, also interferes with the liver's ability to remove excess estrogen and cortisol from your system, thereby failing to short-circuit the vicious cycle of estrogen dominance.

A secondary effect of stress on the body that applies to fat retention in the estrogen dominance scenario occurs with the increased secretion of the hormone prolactin. Increased levels of prolactin, caused by stress, suppress the production of progesterone, allowing the effects of estrogen to increase.

Remember what I said about you doing most of this stuff to yourself? Now you're understanding a little better how your actions and eating habits open the floodgates to counterproductive hormonal activity within your body. The laws of nature demand you either correct this flow by eating the foods your body demands or suffer the consequences.

A woman caught in the vicious estrogen dominance/adrenal fatigue cycle will always feel tired and on edge. It is possible to break this cycle of fatigue by simply giving your body what it needs to operate in the way it was designed to. That will help you ward off the ill effects of stressors on your body. You wouldn't give an auto mechanic the tools of a carpenter and expect them to fix your transmission, would you? So why deprive your body of the "tools" it needs? We will discuss proper eating habits a little later in this book.

While it may be easier for you to visualize the effect estrogen dominance has on women, it affects men as well. There may be some internal mechanisms that affect the estrogen levels in men, but external variables cause men problems in this area to a greater degree.

Chapter Twenty-Two

Xenoestrogens From the Environment

Whether we are discussing men, women, children, or animals, it is the xenoestrogens in our environment that affect us most often and in the most robust manner. These are chemicals from a variety of sources that we encounter every day and throughout each day.

Xenoestrogens mimic estrogen and simulate the biological effects of estrogen. Only a small amount of xenoestrogens must be absorbed before their effects are seen. To make matters worse, these compounds are non-biodegradable, so they stay in the environment for long periods of time.

Xenoestrogens appear to be more potent in expressing estrogen-like effects on your body than do naturally occurring estrogen. What all of this means is that this stuff is out there just waiting to cause you problems.

These chemicals are fat soluble so they can be absorbed through your skin. Such chemicals will accumulate in the fatty tissues of your body and in the fatty tissues of animals that later become the meat in your diet. Once the xenoestrogens are in your body, they stay there for long periods of time.

When you are exposed to xenoestrogens, you pass the estrogen-mimicking effects to your offspring. These chemicals have a powerful effect on the ovaries and testes of your offspring when they are embryos.

Prolonged exposure to xenoestrogens can cause decreased progesterone production in females (and its associated lack of ovulation, leading to infertility) as well as decreased production of sperm in males. Is infertility on the rise as is being reported in the popular media or is it just receiving more media attention? That's a good question without a simple answer.

You must realize that since xenoestrogens are fat soluble and non-biodegradable, they will stay in you and your children for a long, long time. Unless you take steps to reduce the amount of xenoestrogens in your body, you may set your children up for health problems throughout their lives.

It has been well established that the initial signs of puberty are, on average, seen two years earlier than they were forty years ago. The most likely candidate for the early onset of puberty is an increased number of xenoestrogens from the environment finding their way into people's bodies.

To take a little broader outlook, the World Health Organization has reported that breast cancer has become the most common cancer among women throughout the world.

Is it coincidental that the growing number of materials containing xenoestrogens coincides with the rising incidence of breast cancer? Do the increases in xenoestrogens have anything to do with the increases in global populations with an unhealthy accumulation of fat in their bodies? Do these parallels sound scary? They are. Denying these issues will not help you. These environmental threats are something you must deal with to stay healthy in this modern world.

Animals reflect changes in their environment. There have been several identifiable changes to animals caused by xenoestrogen exposure.

Animal behavior and physiology in the wild acts as an early indicator of changes in the environment. With xenoestrogens, the changes in the physiology of animals are striking. Male birds, for example, are exhibiting feminization of their reproductive organs.

In male alligators, researchers are finding abnormally high estrogen levels. These high levels of estrogenic hormones are causing small penis sizes and low levels of testosterone in male alligators. Other creatures such as turtles, fish, and mollusks have undergone gender "reassignment" due to environmentally induced hormonal changes.

All of this begs the question, "Are these types of changes occurring in humans as well?" After all, we live in this polluted world along with the animals. The answer is, yes, signs of environmentally induced estrogen dominance are being found in humans. Increases in prostate, cervical, and breast cancers may be because of xenoestrogens affecting estrogen dominance in humans.

In men, there has been a fifty percent decrease in individual sperm count since 1938 as well as finding undersized penises in boys born to women who were exposed to PCBs. Polychlorinated biphenyls (PCBs) are highly carcinogenic chemical compounds used in industrial and consumer products. United States federal law banned their production in 1978 and by the Stockholm Convention on Persistent Organic Pollutants in 2001. PCBs contain xenohormones that, when ingested or breathed in through the lungs, exert estrogen-like effects on the human body.

Where do these things come from? Before being banned, they were found in many pesticides, solvents, plastics, glues, adhesives, and many other common commercial and household items like cleaners. Once released into the environment, these compounds hang around, as we have already discussed. They're everywhere, or so it seems.

Some of these xenohormones can stop or retard the liver's ability to break down and excrete excess estrogen. Why is this important? Because if the liver cannot break down and get rid of the excess estrogen, it continues to circulate in your bloodstream and do its insidious damage. Or it's stored in fat just to get it out of circulation. This latter method may sound like a solution but storing excess estrogen in body fat simply keeps it in your system longer.

Since excess estrogen, or substances that exert estrogen-like effects, cause both fat and/or water retention, it is important to our discussion concerning unhealthy accumulation of body fat.

The effects of xenoestrogens are rampant in men and women all around the world today. These chemicals may be a contributing factor to the rising rate of unhealthy levels of accumulated body fat around the world. But how does excessive estrogen cause an unhealthy accumulation of this fat?

Chapter Twenty-Three

Estrogen and Fat Accumulation

An unhealthy accumulation of body fat is not just due to overeating or eating the wrong foods. And it has very little to do with willpower alone. Let's take a few minutes to discuss the effect estrogen has on the creation and accumulation of body fat.

Estrogen is made in fatty tissues. This suggests that obesity is a leading cause of estrogen dominance. This is a very significant statement, so let's repeat it and let it sink in. Obesity is a leading cause of estrogen dominance because estrogen is made in fatty tissues. In other words, the more fat your body is storing, the more estrogen your body is producing.

OK, so what?

This is important because estrogen increases fat storage within the body. Fat makes estrogen and then estrogen turns around and stores more fat.

If the relationship between estrogen and body fat is sounding like a self-perpetuating cycle, then you're seeing the big picture. Just like a nuclear reactor gone wild, this cycle will continue until your body suffers from a "meltdown." This meltdown will cause an unhealthy accumulation of body fat and many other undesirable consequences.

Besides making more fat, excess estrogen also inhibits thyroid function. This thyroid dysfunction mimics hypothyroidism, a condition whereby thyroid function is below its normally expected level. How many of you are taking a synthetic thyroid supplement because poor thyroid function is blamed for you retaining body fat?

Many folks began taking thyroid medication because of lack of energy (fatigue), gain in weight, or other symptoms commonly associated with hypothyroidism… even though your thyroid tests were normal.

Estrogen dominance reduces the thyroid's ability to operate properly and is an enormous factor contributing to an unhealthy accumulation of body fat. Estrogen and your thyroid are made to work against each other. While estrogen works to store your food energy as fat, the thyroid should be trying to increase your body's burning of fat for energy use.

When there is an imbalance between estrogen and thyroid hormones, there is, in effect, an imbalance in the utilization of the food energy you consume. What a crummy thing to have happen! And the bad part is that you did not have a clue this was occurring.

The bottom line is that estrogen dominance increases the amount of fat your body stores. Period.

But the problem does not stop here. With increased fat storage comes increasing estrogen production, remember? The result is that you are now firmly ensconced in a vicious cycle of estrogen production and fat storage.

This isn't just a problem for women. Given that xenoestrogens are often absorbed from the environment and stored in body fat, they pose significant risks to both genders.

Some xenoestrogens stop or at least slow down the ability of the liver to break down and excrete excess estrogen, and this only adds to the mess.

Such a cycle looks something like this.

Xenoestrogens cause liver overload which leads to estrogen dominance. Estrogen dominance is what begins the vicious cycle of fat storage. Estrogen decreases thyroid function causing sluggish metabolism which in turn increases estrogen dominance. The dominance of estrogen in your body increases fat storage and as more fat is stored it begins making more estrogen. Thus, the perpetuation of the estrogen dominance/increased fat storage cycle.

Estrogen dominance leads to water retention (another factor associated with not looking slim and trim and leading to things like high blood pressure) and cravings for simple carbohydrates. Simple carbohydrates are found in foods that contain white (refined) sugar, white (refined) flour, white (not whole grain) rice, and pastas made from refined flours.

Nothing is more appealing than a sugary pastry made with these simple carbohydrates when you have a craving for something to eat. It should now make sense why you have cravings and are putting on weight all out of proportion to what you are eating regardless of how much you exercise.

Chapter Twenty-Four

Unhealthy Weight Retention and Cortisol

Estrogen dominance is one problem. Another sinister scenario occurs with the stress hormone, cortisol. Everything we've been discussing leads to an unhealthy accumulation of body fat, which leads to insulin resistance, a condition where blood sugar cannot be satisfactorily used by the body's cells, thereby increasing the levels of glucose in the blood, leading to Type II diabetes. This sequence of events places excess stress on the adrenal glands and increases cortisol levels, which deposits more fat around the belly. Which, in turn… well, you get the idea.

Such a sequence looks something like this.

An unhealthy accumulation of body fat leads to increased insulin resistance. That results in increased blood glucose which is known as diabetes. Diabetes increases stress on the adrenal glands leading to increased cortisol and more fat accumulation around the belly. That increase in unwanted body fat begins the entire vicious cycle all over again.

Is the fatty tissue around your belly the only place fat is deposited? How about in the liver itself?

Do you remember reading how an unhealthy body fat accumulation can lead to insulin resistance, which leads to a fatty liver? The liver not only breaks down excess estrogen, but also excess cortisol. How then do you think having a fatty liver and a compromised ability to break down and excrete excess estrogen and cortisol will affect you?

Yes. You guessed it.

The result of these cycles perpetuating themselves is that you have many vicious cycles going on all at once. Some cycles operate independently of one another while others feed off, or magnify the effects of, each other. Regardless of how you look at it, an unhealthy accumulation of body fat results in a self-perpetuating catastrophe, and this calamity wreaks havoc on your body.

Your body's organs and systems work together as cooperating elements to protect your body from harm. When one unit falters, all the other units are affected, either directly or indirectly, but the result is the same. You become fat and unhealthy.

It's also easy to see how increased cortisol and estrogen dominance work together to store more fat. When stored fat then turns around and makes more estrogen and cortisol, it magnifies the effects.

Did you ever wonder why people always seem to get fatter and fatter as time goes on? This may be the reason dieting, normal amounts of exercise, and heaps of willpower are never enough to allow you or a loved one to achieve a more normal amount of body fat.

It may appear there is no way out of these vicious cycles because the liver is the primary organ responsible for breaking down and excreting estrogen, but this isn't entirely true. There is a way to cast off the chains of these fat producing cycles.

You can detoxify your liver so it is once again capable of breaking down excess estrogen and cortisol. Now, let's look more closely at how to break these cycles of fat production.

Chapter Twenty-Five

Breaking the Cycles

We will get into how to speed up the process of stopping these fat-producing cycles in the next chapter but a good place to start is by eating fresh fruits and raw vegetables so your liver has the enzymes it needs to break down estrogen and cortisol. Throw in a little exercise to keep the body functioning the way it is supposed to and avoid xenoestrogen-containing substances as much as possible. Especially avoid things like birth control pills, which, in addition to raising estrogen levels, have been found to reduce the level of antioxidants in the liver.

Birth control pills put significant stress on the liver, both directly and indirectly. For example, many oral contraceptives lower the amount of the antioxidant known as glutathione in the liver. Glutathione is believed to decrease the risk of liver damage from common chemicals and medications, so decreasing the concentration of this antioxidant puts your liver at greater risk for toxic damage. If the liver is damaged, it cannot break down and excrete excess estrogen. That puts you into estrogen dominance, which... UH-OH! There's that vicious cycle again!

Can estrogen dominance be reduced just by making a few, minor, healthier lifestyle changes? Is it really so easy to avoid estrogen dominance and an unhealthy accumulation of unwanted body fat? Yes, it is.

Women who eat a diet rich in plants, like fresh fruits and raw vegetables, are less likely to experience symptoms related to estrogen dominance. That's not too hard to do, right? Isn't it simple?

It is simple! And yet most people don't do it. Why?

This is a totally reasonable question to ask yourself. Only your health and the health of successive generations are in the balance. No big deal, right?

Wrong.

The first step in avoiding estrogen dominance is to reduce your exposure to xenoestrogen-containing contaminants as much as possible. This is easier said than done simply because xenoestrogens are pervasive in the products you encounter every day. Because xenoestrogens are incredibly stable and do not break down easily, we cannot combat this problem simply by banning all xenoestrogen-containing products. There is already an unhealthy buildup up of xenoestrogens in the environment that won't just disappear.

Considering that xenoestrogens are found in many of the products you currently use or are exposed to daily (carpet and home furnishings, as well as auto emissions come to mind), how are you to avoid them all? The simple answer is that you can't. You can't control every environmental factor. You can, however, prepare for the worst and hope for the best.

What you can do is make sure your liver works properly and continues to do so. True, this is only an alternative to complete xenoestrogen eradication, but it is workable and will help protect you and your children from estrogen dominance.

Besides supplying your body with essential enzymes and phytonutrients to increase liver function, eating fruits and vegetables will have additional positive effects on your health. The added fiber these foodstuffs contain will make you feel satiated with less food so you may lose some weight because you'll be eating less. Just as important, the added fiber in your diet will help "hide" some xenoestrogens that find their way into your gut until they can be eliminated.

By trapping xenoestrogens in a slurry of fiber passing through your gut they will have less of a chance of coming into direct contact with the intestinal wall and being absorbed. Hopefully, by traveling within a slurry of fiber so they cannot be absorbed by your body, the xenoestrogens will continue through your entire digestive tract until you excrete them.

Eating organically grown food also helps. The fact that organic foods have more nutrients than those grown conventionally is important. Besides, when foods are grown in nutrition and mineral-depleted soils more xenoestrogen containing fertilizers and pesticides must be used to cultivate them. Eating organically grown foods will eliminate one chemical source of xenoestrogens, specifically, those found on the surface of and inside the produce you consume.

Xenoestrogens may also work themselves into your diet indirectly. They often feed livestock chemically treated grain containing xenoestrogens. The xenoestrogens are then stored in the animal's fat, which is consumed by you as meat.

To avoid this type of xenoestrogen contamination, it's best to eat organic meat, such as grass-fed beef or free-range chicken.

So, to wrap this up, thyroid problems, insulin problems, sluggish liver function, poor nutritional habits, hormone imbalances, dangerously cultivated food, and environmental poisons and toxins all enter the equation that ultimately determines whether you develop a healthy or an unhealthy body habitus (body habitus means physique or body build).

When you eat the proper foods and get a little exercise, you will be healthier and slimmer. General good health and being slim go together.

However, when you get healthier and slimmer, you must have a realistic outlook on what being healthy and slim means TO YOU.

Don't expect to look like the young models in the fashion magazines if your genes are not designed to express themselves in that way. You're probably like most of us and you live in the real world, so be practical when setting goals and expectations. Relax and enjoy your health and life. It's worth it.

Chapter Twenty-Six

Pollution, Overload, and Detoxification

So, if the environmental pollutants don't kill you, your leaky gut will, right?

Wrong.

It's your liver to the rescue! Unless, of course, your liver is overloaded and unable to process toxins and excrete them properly. Then you're in a dangerous situation. Well, not really, but you must take decisive action or you're going to have a snowball effect of problems heading your way. At least you still have a chance to avoid more problems by doing something about it while you can.

Exactly what role does the liver play in all of this and why should you be concerned about it?

If the gut is leaking bad stuff into the bloodstream, the liver must work overtime to remove these toxins.

How long do you think it will take for your liver to become overworked, overloaded, and unable to keep up with the excess load being placed upon it? Not long at all.

There are only a finite number of blood purifying tasks the liver can accomplish at any given time, and they are limited by several factors. When the sheer volume of toxins overcomes the liver pushing it past its ability to handle the deluge of toxins being dumped into it, strange things happen.

Toxin overload results in the inability of the liver to filter contaminants out of the blood, so contaminants continue circulating in the bloodstream, which causes a lot of problems. These are toxic substances your body is supposed to get rid of as quickly as possible, but that cannot happen when there is an overabundance of them entering your body at such a rapid rate.

The liver stores and filters your blood, removing toxins and infectious organisms by processing approximately three pints of blood every minute. Can you now understand why the liver is known as the "oil filter of the body?"

Most blood is carried to the liver via the portal vein, directly from the gut. Blood from the gut carries nutrients and toxins to the liver so the toxins can be detoxified.

The liver is the primary organ responsible for the detoxification of most of the toxins entering your body. If a leaky gut is involved, the volume of toxins entering your body increases exponentially.

If your liver is operating at peak proficiency, and there are no excessive amounts of toxins entering your body, the liver can handle its detoxification functions handily under normal circumstances. However, if a leaky gut is dumping harmful toxins into your bloodstream, the liver quickly becomes overloaded and unable to keep up with the massive volume.

There can be several stages, or phases, within the liver, where the liver fails in its job of removing toxins from the body. Let's take a moment to outline what they are and where problems can arise.

Chapter Twenty-Seven

Detoxifying Your Liver

Let's review a bit since it has been a while since we covered this. The process of liver detoxification is composed of two phases, Phase I and Phase II.

Phase I detoxification directly neutralizes many toxic chemicals. Those it doesn't directly neutralize get converted into intermediate chemicals. These intermediate chemicals can be more toxic than the original toxin they were derived from. However, if Phase II of liver detoxification works properly, the intermediate chemicals are immediately rendered harmless, then converted into a form that can be excreted through the kidneys in urine or via bile to be expelled in the feces.

While up to seventy-five percent of the detoxification activity takes place in the liver, some takes place in other tissues such as the wall of the intestines. The role of the digestive tract and the friendly gut bacteria living there were discussed briefly when we covered the Leaky Gut Syndrome. These bacteria can produce compounds that directly aid in detoxification.

Both phases of detoxification taking place in the liver have unique characteristics. However, it is essential they function in balance with each other. This minimizes intermediate chemicals from lingering around so the detoxification process can be completed efficiently.

Intermediate chemicals cannot be excreted until they go through Phase II. Depletion of nutrients necessary for normal functioning of

Phase II detoxification can cause a build-up of intermediate chemicals created in Phase I.

A steady supply of sulfur containing amino acids or inorganic sulfate from the diet is necessary for continuing Phase II operation. Fasting, or consumption of high amounts of acetaminophen, for example, may deplete the amount of sulfate and inhibit the entire detoxification process. Does that make it easier to understand how taking medications, whether prescribed or over the counter, can affect bodily processes in ways we don't normally know about?

There may even be a genetic component determining an individual's ability to detoxify chemicals. Have you ever wondered why members of the same family are overweight? Of course, it can be many factors, but we should not ignore the possibility of them having an inability to rapidly detoxify pollutants.

There is also evidence metabolic conditions such as insulin-dependent diabetes and obesity can lead to changes in the detoxification process.

That's rather interesting, isn't it?

A vicious cycle of obesity and insulin-dependent diabetes causes liver detoxification problems, which leads to more obesity and diabetes. There are numerous vicious cycles implicated in many serious conditions when the inability of the liver to detoxify toxins is considered.

Vicious cycles occurring because of disruptions in liver functioning are self-perpetuating and will continue creating havoc within the body until the cycle is broken. Assuring the liver can efficiently detoxify pollution and toxins demolishes these vicious cycles and stops them from putting fat on what should be your svelte frame.

You want to keep a steady supply of antioxidants in your body to keep the detoxification process operating smoothly. This combats the free radicals forming in the intermediary stage between Phase I and

Phase II. If these free radicals are not stopped, secondary tissue damage can result. You really do not want that to happen.

An example of intermediate chemicals that cause tissue damage if a sufficient amount of antioxidants are not present can be found in the polycylic hydrocarbons you will get from cigarette smoke and char-broiled meats.

Both Phase I and Phase II detoxification processes depend on enzymes that must be supplied through dietary sources that are consumed daily. Where do enzymes come from? Enzymes mainly come from eating raw vegetables. Can you now see why it is important to eat your vegetables like your mother and grandmother told you to do? And you can't substitute cooked vegetables for raw as cooking destroys many, if not all, of the essential enzymes.

We need phytonutrients in both Phase I and Phase II of the detoxification system and several promising studies show phytonutrients lower the risk of certain cancers. So, they are important.

Eat your raw vegetables. They are a mandatory part of your daily diet, and this is not negotiable. It must be done if you ever hope to have your liver operate properly to allow you to lose weight.

The research pertaining to an individual's ability to detoxify toxins has significantly increased the clinical understanding of the detoxification process. Some studies show impaired detoxification may play a significant role in lupus erythematosus and rheumatoid arthritis. Further research will have to be done to determine to what extent flaws in the detoxification process are pertinent to these and other disease processes. But why wait? Clean up your liver's detoxification process today and you'll never know how many terrible health problems you can avoid.

Chapter Twenty-Eight

Knowledge is Power

Detoxification of the liver, or purification as it is also known, is a process that puts a significant burden on the body. Therefore, a highly refined source of nutrients is necessary, and it is up to you to assure your body is getting what it needs when it needs it. You really should know all the ins and outs of how your body handles the detoxification of toxins because your preconceived notions as to what is good for you may not be true.

For example, juice or water fasting may be detrimental to your body's ability to detoxify and excrete toxins. Such fasting results in the breakdown of muscle since the body needs a constant flow of amino acids (which come from proteins and muscle is made of protein). If amino acids are not forthcoming from your diet, your body will use its own protein reserves. That means your own body will cannibalize your muscles. That is a bad thing to have happen and should be avoided because juice or water fasting does not provide protein to meet your daily needs.

It has been shown that water fasting by laboratory animals (a "diet" in which no food and only water is consumed for an extended period) made them more susceptible to the effects of toxins. Other types of fasting results in Phase I becoming too active in the manufacture of harmful metabolites to the point of Phase II not being able to keep up. An overload of newly manufactured metabolites from Phase I, as stated previously, is usually very detrimental to the body.

Once again, with dietary schemes such as water fasting, know what you are doing before you do harm to yourself. It would be a sorry irony if you try to be conscientious of your health and cause more damage.

However, a large quantity of pure water is needed to wash the water-soluble metabolized toxins from the body, so make sure you are consuming enough along with a well-balanced diet. That means pure water. Not tap water with a bunch of chemicals in it. Use bottled spring water or purified water.

There are several water purifiers on the market that do a very credible job, especially the units using a process called reverse osmosis. Read up on the subject and be an educated consumer because there are some unscrupulous vendors out there selling pure junk. Don't lose your money and your health just because you are too cheap to buy the good water purifiers or, worse yet, are too lazy to research the subject thoroughly.

An excellent source of protein is also essential for a detoxification program as it supplies needed amino acids that are essential to the detoxification process. Meat is still the easiest way to get enough protein into your diet. If you do not eat meat, things become more difficult to assure you get these vital nutrients into your system.

We need an excellent source of energy to perform a proper detoxification procedure. Fats supply energy for detoxification, but only certain fats.

Long-chain fats can cause problems for those with Leaky Gut Syndrome. Therefore, medium-chain triglycerides such as olive oil are an excellent source of fat to consume for energy. Not only is olive oil absorbed in the small intestine without the presence of bile from the liver, but it is also known to be helpful to those suffering from malabsorption syndromes. Olive oil has been shown to be supportive of the liver, which is important since the liver is being compelled to perform more toxin excreting functions.

Chapter Twenty-Nine

Permanent Lifestyle Changes

This is the bottom line. The rest of this book gave you some great supportive information and background you must understand, but this is the key aspect.

If you want to rejuvenate your liver, then do the steps that are necessary; let me repeat that, NECESSARY for you to maintain the excretory pathways within your liver. Then you will achieve your goal of maintaining a healthier amount of body fat for life.

By normalizing the excretory functions of your liver, it will correctly regulate the food energy you take into your body. You will see changes in your eating habits you developed over years or even decades. Usually, you've developed those eating habits based on what tastes good and you're in the mood for at the moment without putting any serious thought into what foods you're eating or in what amounts you are consuming them.

When your liver is operating correctly, and your body is properly nourished, your urge to overeat will be curbed while your food cravings will be reduced or eliminated. You will know when you are truly "full" and ready to stop eating instead of waiting until you're stuffed and can barely move.

To learn some neat tricks and tips on how to achieve all these wonderful things see my book *The Psychology Behind Eating: Scientifically Proven Mind Games to Lose Weight and Keep It Off*. In the psychology behind eating book, I offer solutions to what you can do to adapt your lifestyle and temperament toward food to naturally maintain a slimmer, healthier body.

But for now, let's discuss how you can get your liver operating correctly so it will do all these wondrous things for you.

First, you must fix your Leaky Gut Syndrome if that is a problem for you. This situation must be addressed first because a leaking gut, if present, will place an astronomical amount of stress on the liver and overload it.

If you suffer from such a syndrome, you will need to heal your entire digestive system. Yes, I know this is more than you bargained for, but it is reality. You either give your body what it needs to operate correctly, or you will suffer the consequences of ill health and an unhealthy accumulation of body fat for the rest of your life. The choice is yours. Choose well to live a healthy, happier life.

Only after fixing your leaking gut will you be able to get your overloaded liver functioning correctly. As discussed in the chapter about Leaky Gut Syndrome, you should seek the help of a healthcare professional trained in nutritional therapies. Their expertise will be invaluable to you.

After fixing your leaking gut, you can then use a liver detoxification program to improve the functioning of your liver. We will discuss a few of the liver detoxification programs available so you can determine what may work best for you. There are many more available, but these few will give you the basics. You will have the information you need to go off on your own to explore other avenues of achieving the same goal if you so desire.

The liver detoxification programs reviewed in this book are not being endorsed as the only solutions, but I know these work. We will explore several programs so you can decide which will best fit your needs and desires. One is not necessarily better than the others, just different.

If you choose to do other detoxification programs, you are on your own to determine if they are suitable for your needs. Just be aware there is some real junk out there being peddled as liver detoxification products. Buyer beware.

When pursuing your own detoxification program, there are a few things that you must remember:

- You cannot eat the sheer volume of foods that are packed into nutritional supplements, so supplements will help you achieve your goal more quickly.

- Organically grown foods have higher nutritive value than those grown non-organically.

- Good quality fresh foods are not available year-round in many parts of the world due to changing seasons, but nutritional supplements usually are.

Organically grown, whole food nutritional supplements, made by a reputable company that has been in business for decades, are the way to go for most of us. Supplements are easy to take, convenient, nutritionally balanced, and have been formulated and quality checked by biochemists for nutritional value. Supplements are the "fast food" of the healthy eating world, and supplements fit your lifestyle year-round, regardless of where you live.

Please remember that raw vegetables will be the basis of your new style of eating. This is not because it is "rabbit food" that will keep you slim due to the lack of calories found in such foods. Rather, it is the enzymes and phytonutrients found in raw vegetables that you need daily for your liver to maintain correct operation.

Eating raw vegetables is non-negotiable. Without these enzymes and phytonutrients, taken in sufficient amounts every day, you will always have an unhealthy accumulation of unwanted body fat. Period.

It's easy for critics to say that anyone eating raw vegetables as a large portion of their daily diet will lose weight. And that's true. However, observed changes in the symptoms you recorded prior to beginning this program will prove that significant changes are occurring within your body. When those symptoms disappear or reduce in intensity, they become your personal "canary."

Let me take a moment here to explain that the concept of a "Canary in The Mineshaft" is explained in much greater detail in my book *Foods Making You Fat, Unhealthy, and Unhappy: Your Personal Roadmap to Fix Problems Doctors Cannot.* It is an important concept to grasp.

Discovering your personal "canaries" is what gives you the information you need to determine if you are falling back into your old eating habits. If you are, you can make corrections before you gain back the weight you lost.

There are no blanket statements that can be made about how you are supposed to eat. Everyone is a unique individual and your body demands specific foods that work with it. Conversely, you must avoid the foods that work against it. That's why we will go through an extensive process (extensive, but easy, you'll see) to determine your canaries.

Canaries are a fun and whimsical concept I came up with that is based upon monitoring the symptoms you are suffering from and then see which ones disappear or reduce in intensity after you make the correct dietary changes your individual body demands.

If you revert to your old eating habits, these canary symptoms will reappear to remind you in very certain terms that you must get back to the foods your body demands. That will keep you looking great, feeling tremendous, and being the best you've ever been.

Canaries were designed to be fun and whimsical, but they are very serious tools we can use to keep ourselves on the right track regardless of whether our goal is to keep weight off after we lose it, look as young and vibrant as possible, or to improve our outlook on life. Of course, you can do all three, and your personal canaries will help you do it.

The information in the *Foods Making You Fat, Unhealthy, and Unhappy: Your Personal Roadmap to Fix Problems Doctors Cannot* book makes it easy to choose the right foods for you, since you have distinctive dietary needs when compared to everyone else. It takes you through a step-by-step process to determine which foods you should eat, and which ones are detrimental to you.

Eating the wrong foods can cause several symptoms (some of which are so strange you would never guess they are related to what you have been eating simply because they are the wrong foods for you). Until you go through the process of determining which foods you personally should eat and which ones to avoid, you will just be guessing. That could jeopardize not only your ability to lose weight but also any hope you have of living a better, more symptom free life.

As you go through the process of discovering which foods your body wants (which makes it thrive) and the foods it does not want (which will give you some sign it is not happy with those foods) you will want to make two lists. One list will be of the foods you should eat, and the other list is those foods you should avoid. Keep these lists in a safe place. Make a few copies of them and stash them in different places because you will refer to them often as you create or modify recipes using the foods that will make your body thrive.

I had to write additional books covering the science and psychology behind eating and weight loss because there was just too much information to put into a single book. The knowledge found in these books encompasses decades of research by the top scientists in their fields of study. Besides, the quantity of information is much more understandable if you read it in smaller, more manageable bits.

For right now, just remember that your "canaries" are the symptoms you suffered from before beginning your liver detoxification program and will continue monitoring as a warning that things are recurring so you can take corrective action. Avoiding an unwanted accumulation of body fat from reappearing can easily be avoided if you monitor your canaries. Waiting until you get to the other books in this series is well worth the delay.

Chapter Thirty

Professional Health Care Strongly Advised

You should seek the help of a healthcare professional with an extensive education in nutritional therapies. We discussed the wide variety of healthcare professionals previously who may be involved with nutritional therapies.

Unfortunately, most of these practitioners do not fall under a single title, so they are sometimes difficult to find. You may have to find them via word of mouth and referrals from your family or friends. An Internet search may also help find ones in your area. However, functional medicine doctors are usually medical doctors with specialized training, and they are the easiest to find with an Internet search.

There are many different types of healthcare professionals who are carrying the burden of bringing true nutritional counseling to the American public. To make our discussion about them easier, we will simply refer to them all as functional medicine doctors even though most are not medical doctors.

A functional medicine doctor uses a biology-based systems approach (like what we have been discussing) to identify and address the root cause (or causes) of disease because they recognize the importance of offering an individualized approach to the causes of disease.

Even some large healthcare institutions are offering functional medicine. For example, in 2014 Cleveland Clinic was the first academic medical center in the country to establish a dedicated functional medicine program, so this is not some far out new healthcare discipline you should be leery about trusting your health to.

It's a good idea to be under the care of a health care professional while undergoing detoxification or making any major lifestyle changes. If the truth were known, most of you have grave health conditions that need attending to before serious and possibly irreversible conditions present themselves.

Whether it is only a mildly irritating condition or whether it is a serious "on-your-way-to-the-grave" situation, you need nutritional counseling. A knowledgeable healthcare professional can help guide you toward better health for the long haul.

For example, some of the Nutri-West products we will be discussing in one of the protocols you may choose to use for liver detoxification have herbs in them. Herbs are nothing more than mild, naturally occurring drugs. There is the possibility of complications if prescription medication is being taken. These are rare situations as the number of interactions is small, but you should be under the care of a qualified healthcare practitioner to learn about these potential problems. The good side is once you consume the proper nutritional supplements and clean up your lifestyle, you might get off the expensive prescription medications you are currently taking.

Think about this for a moment. It is not a hard concept to understand.

Coordinate any discontinuation of medication with your medical doctor. Never stop taking prescribed medication without professional consultation.

There are good reasons you should be under a health care professional's care as you undertake any lifestyle changes. While there are no reported interactions with drugs, combinations of nutrients may have blood-thinning compounds that could thin the blood too much if taken in combination with medications such as Coumadin or aspirin. Not all doctors are schooled in using nutritional supplements. Remember our discussion at the beginning of this book? Heed the advice of the health care professional that has completed extensive study in these subjects.

The other side of the coin is if you consume a combination of nutrients containing blood thinning compounds like fish oil, you may not need Coumadin or aspirin to keep your blood thin.

Most folks do not realize that proper nutrients and diet can reduce potentially serious health-threatening conditions. Proper nutrition addresses many of the reasons people suffer strokes, heart attacks, or other serious health problems.

To illustrate this, one technique I've used over the years is to refer my patients for carotid artery ultra-sound tests performed to determine the amount of plaque formation in their carotid arteries. Repeated testing one year later should show reduced plaque formation if they have truly adopted a proper diet and nutritional regimen. It is their poor dietary habits that get them in trouble and correct eating habits get them out of it.

The American mindset of waiting until a heart attack and/or stroke occurs before improving a person's habits is ludicrous and expensive. It is predicated on the assumption you will survive unscathed and then have time to improve your eating habits.

Eat properly, be healthier and slimmer to try avoiding the expense and emotional trauma of a heart attack or stroke. You should put at least as much effort into caring for your health as you do to maintain your car.

On the upside, most of what we are discussing may help you regain your health so you will not have to take liver overloading drugs. That is why I will repeat myself and state that you should let your medical doctor know what you are doing so they can monitor your medications and physical condition.

Previously, we used the example of where your high blood pressure normalizes because you regained your health. In this instance, you certainly do not want to artificially drive it below normal with the use of high blood pressure medications that are no longer needed.

Whatever condition you may be seeing your medical doctor for, you will want to let them know what you are doing so they can monitor it for you. When you go through the process of streamlining your eating habits you will see changes, some of them major changes, that take place.

This is especially true if you follow the process I've written about in the book *Foods Making You Fat, Unhealthy, and Unhappy: Your Personal Roadmap to Fix Problems Doctors Cannot.* You will see health conditions disappear that you thought you'd have for your entire life. Do the smart thing and coordinate your efforts to improve your health with your doctor.

It's important to remember there's a lot more to health than just being slim. Now, let's look at a few of the liver detoxification programs I am familiar with and have used successfully.

Chapter Thirty-One

Standard Process's Detoxification Program

Standard Process's Detox Balance program was developed to be a gentle liver detoxification experience. The importance of being gentle cannot be underestimated.

There are many liver detoxification programs that have been available over the years. This includes gall bladder flushes. These types of flushes have been rather "brisk." While they may have worked to a certain extent, they usually work too well and too quickly, giving people undesirable symptoms. Therein lies the problem with older detoxification programs that have not been well researched and may not be based upon well-established science.

Think about this for a minute. The liver is overloaded with toxins and functions below par. Therefore, toxins have been stored in the fatty tissues of your body or are floating around in your bloodstream. If you start a liver detoxification program that is rapidly going to liberate all those toxins, you will get very sick and likely give up on the entire process. Rapid liberation of toxins affects all systems of the body, and the results are not pleasant.

That's exactly what would happen with the older detoxification programs. It was worth it in the long run, but why suffer flu-like symptoms if you don't have to? Standard Process's program slowly releases toxins from the body and limits unpleasant effects.

The goal of gentle detoxification is why the Standard Process (SP) program doesn't allow you to have lemon or avocado while performing liver detoxification. These foods thin the bile, which would increase the "dumping" of toxins from the liver.

The liver produces bile that is stored in the gallbladder. Bile contains toxins. If the bile is released into the small intestine too quickly, it will release toxins along with the bile. A rapid release of the toxin contaminated bile into the small intestine will make you feel bad when the toxins are reabsorbed by the small intestine and dumped into the bloodstream. It is for reasons like this one that you should use an established program based on science and years of experience.

I consider the SP program to be a "moderate" detoxification program because it allows you to eat fresh fruit up to fifty percent of the total volume of vegetables you are eating. That's a lot.

It's much more appetizing for Americans to eat fresh fruit than it is to eat raw vegetables. The typical American is used to sweet foods and fresh fruit supplies sugars. Even though sugars are natural and contained in a high fiber fruit, fruit is more palatable to most folks than are vegetables.

However, too much fruit compared to the total volume of raw vegetables contains too many calories and you won't lose weight, assuming that is your goal. If you are consuming too many calories from fruit, your body will not need to burn fat for energy. The result is you will not lose weight. That's no fun! So, eat lots of raw vegetables. You'll be glad you did.

Also, if you are not burning fat, the toxins stored in body fat will remain there. You really want to lose the fat and the toxins stored within it. If you are going to use the program, you may as well reap all the benefits.

Before discussing the program, let's define what you are trying to accomplish.

Detoxification is also known as purification or cleansing. It is the process by which the body cleanses itself of toxins (poisons). The liver, digestive tract (gut), kidneys, bladder, lymphatic system, lungs, and skin are the major systems and organs involved with this process.

The SP program supports the liver and colon nutritionally, as this is the elimination pathway most advantageous for the body to use. That makes sense since the liver, via the bile and gallbladder, dumps toxins into the small intestines. Since toxins are now in the gut tube, it is easiest to just expel them with your next bowel movement.

If you often have trouble with having an easy, regular bowel movement (BM) you will be pleasantly surprised because this program often helps with that problem. When you have easier BMs while on any of the detoxification programs, please write it down as one of your "canaries" so you can monitor it as time goes on. If it recurs regularly, you must look at getting our liver fully functioning again. It is easy to have these problems sneak back on you because of your daily exposure to environmental pollutants. Besides, bowel movements are one of the easiest symptoms to monitor and are a bodily function you want to keep operating correctly throughout your life span.

The liver, gut tube, and kidneys are primary excretory systems. All other organs and systems are secondary elimination pathways. There are problems that result from using these secondary pathways if their use is necessitated in times of crisis, such as when the liver and colon cannot handle an overload of toxins.

As an example, if the skin must be used as an excretory organ, toxins may damage the skin as they exit. This may result in eczema, skin rash, or other conditions. Skin rashes aren't pleasant, so using primary excretory routes via the bowels or kidneys is preferred.

To best accomplish a weight management detoxification program, the process must be gentle and reduce excess fat stores in your body while being high in fiber and low in fat. To lose weight, the amount of energy being used by your body must be more than you are taking in. Your body must tap into your fat reserves and use the energy stored there.

All of this must be accomplished without you losing muscle mass. Therefore, appropriate nutrition must be consumed to avoid the loss of muscle. Once the desired amount of body fat is reached, your food intake must be balanced with the amount of energy used by your body. Healthy liver function is mandatory because the liver controls fat burning.

Let's face reality here for a moment. You did not gain your unhealthy weight overnight and you will not lose it overnight either. Following the completion of whatever liver detoxification program you choose; you should give yourself up to one year to establish a healthy amount of body fat. By that time, you will have adopted a healthier lifestyle so you can maintain your healthier weight with little trouble.

In my office, patients that stayed with the SP detoxification program typically lost between thirteen and seventeen pounds during the initial twenty-one-day program and experienced other physical changes. Note what changes you experience and then monitor them. If they eventually change back to what they were previously, then you know something is amiss and needs to be corrected.

You may notice your frequency and quantity of urination increasing for the first few days while detoxifying your liver. Also, the frequency and quantity of bowel movements may increase. People have forgotten, if they ever knew, how many bowel movements and how much material should be passed in a day. It is an eye-opening experience for many people as well as being a welcome relief.

Occasionally, people will experience flu-like symptoms of headache, generalized aches and pains, itchy skin, or fatigue. This is because their body is very toxic and large quantities of toxins are being released. Extra water and lots of fresh vegetables may make the entire process go more smoothly.

Part way through the program, most people begin feeling much better than they have in years or even decades. Now is the time to identify your "canaries" while they are fresh in your mind. Write them down so you do not forget them! They will be important to monitor later.

You may find you have major nutritional deficiencies that have reduced your body's ability to handle food and food energy efficiently. You may need additional nutritional supplementation to bring your entire digestive system up to par. It may not be just the liver that is in trouble and causing you to accumulate unhealthy amounts of fat in various parts of your body.

Only by nutritionally supporting your stomach and gut tube, including your lower bowels, can you digest and eliminate the food waste and toxins that will move through your digestive system. Other bodily systems that may need attention include the thyroid, adrenal glands, pancreas, and possibly others. These may have all degraded because of the liver overload or they may have been a contributing factor causing liver overload. These are the things your functional medicine doctor can help you identify and correct.

Usually, I suggest fixing your Leaky Gut Syndrome (if present) and then starting a liver detoxification program. Always follow any other suggestions your healthcare professional makes. You will be happy with the resultant newfound health you thought was gone with your youth.

The SP Detox Balance program includes an all-in-one shake that is supported by nutritious meals the company suggests. They make the entire program easy by providing a toxicity questionnaire so you can evaluate any symptoms you have prior to beginning the program and can then reevaluate afterwards. You will also use the symptom list you compiled before beginning any of the suggested interventions.

Standard Process offers both a ten-day program and a twenty-eight-day one. You can choose which you want to try. If you begin with the ten-day program and see positive results, you may eventually use the twenty-eight-day one. Success makes you more willing to do what needs to be done, especially when you see how much better you are feeling.

This is another example of the behavior modification process I describe in the book The *Psychology Behind Eating: Scientifically Proven Mind Games to Lose Weight and Keep It Off*. The information found in this book can help you obtain a healthier lifestyle and slimmer body much more easily.

Why would you choose a twenty-one-day program instead of the shorter ten day one? Well, it's because of the gradual detoxification that takes place under a program dragged out over a longer period. Most of you reading this book are as toxic as a Superfund toxic waste dump. The slower twenty-one-day detoxification process will gently guide you back to a healthier body while reducing the possibility of severe or toxic reactions.

"Use the best and ignore the rest" is a good philosophy to follow in many areas of life and it certainly applies to the area of nutrition. Quality detoxification programs are based on solid medical studies but the do-it-yourself programs you find on the Internet probably are not.

It is vital you not only inform your healthcare practitioner of your present complaints and past medical history, but you will have to give them your current experiences with any dietary changes or modifications while on any of these detoxification programs. Include the positive and the negative so they, and you, will be able to monitor your progress closely.

Most of these programs eliminate sugar and caffeine from your diet. Removing caffeine and sugar from your diet may cause withdrawal headaches, so begin gradually weaning yourself off these items to reduce the severity of symptoms when you cut them out of your diet completely. If you refuse to give these up, you are not going along with the program, and you will not get the results you desire. Period.

These programs require commitment. You must give your body what it needs and keep the stuff that is detrimental to it out of your diet. Remember, these are the rules nature and your body have established. You can either live by those rules or learn to live with the consequences.

If you insist on doing the things that are keeping you fat, you will stay fat. Remember those rules of nature. Play by the rules or give it up. Torturing yourself by fighting a losing battle is ludicrous.

Both the National Cancer Institute and the National Institutes of Health recommend you eat five to nine servings of fresh fruits and vegetables each day. Truthfully, do you get anywhere near these many servings of fresh fruit and vegetables every day? Every week? Truthfully now! Few people do.

To detoxify your liver and restore proper functioning to it, you should eat vegetables and fruits. Yep! Rabbit food! But it's what you need. Then you can add some of your usual foods back into your diet.

It's important for you to return to some of your usual foods. If you could not add some of your favorite foods back into your diet, you will never change your eating habits.

Many people seem to be so enthralled at all the positive health improvements taking place within their body that they stick with the program enthusiastically. It amazes people how good they feel while on programs such as these. They truly surprise themselves. You just need to be patient. We are an impatient bunch and want immediate results, but the body needs time to heal before giving us the results we so desperately desire.

It's encouraged that you eat as many fresh vegetables as you can hold because of the vital enzymes and phytonutrients they provide. There is no limit on vegetables. The more the better. Go for it!

Because of the eat-as-many-vegetables-as-you-want facet of liver detoxification and weight loss, you should never go hungry. Ever.

You must drink at least eight large glasses of water per day, which you should do anyway, but it is imperative during liver detoxification. This is very important because the toxins must be expelled from your body as quickly as possible. The water is not only used in the chemical processes taking place in your body, but it will be lost in urine as it carries the toxins away. You want a lot of urine carrying all those toxins away as soon as possible, so make sure your body has a lot of water to keep things flowing.

Water is also needed to saturate the fiber in the nutritional supplements you will be consuming. If you have a high fiber intake but neglect to drink lots of water, you will think you are passing a brick the next time you go to the bathroom. Drink lots of water to avoid any unpleasant consequences.

I have heard the lame excuse that folks won't drink water because they don't want to spend all day in the restroom. Well, guess what? You're supposed to keep huge amounts of fluid moving through your body. It's the way things are supposed to work, so make sure you give your body what it needs to function the way it was designed to.

Remember those rules of nature? Well, drinking lots of water is another one. Follow it unfailingly.

This is especially important for women. With a shorter urethra than men, women are more susceptible to bacteria traveling up that short tube and giving them a bladder infection. The frequent flow of urine out of the body literally washes bacteria out of the shorter urethra, preventing bladder infections. Cool, huh? All it takes to avoid most bladder infections is to drink enough water every day, all day long. Do it.

You should relieve your bladder seven to twelve times per day. If that is a major inconvenience in your life, you are much too busy.

Good liver detoxification systems work. You just need to follow the simple formulas. But you must follow them exactly as they are designed.

Remember, you are not on a "diet" to lose weight. You are returning function to your liver. It's a medical-type thing. Do it right or don't waste your time and money.

If you needed stitches to close a gash in your arm, you wouldn't ask the doctor to only stitch you up halfway, would you? For the liver detoxification system to be effective, it must be strictly followed otherwise the results will not be optimized.

Remember. I didn't make these rules, nature did. You and I can only play by the rules nature has set forth. If we don't, then we must pay the consequences, and that is not pleasant.

You are only cheating yourself if you cheat on the liver detoxification process. Do yourself a favor. If you are not serious about getting rid of your unhealthy accumulation of body fat, don't torture yourself. If you think a plan like this is too difficult to follow exactly, put this book down, eat anything you want and in any amount. Enjoy yourself if that's what makes you happy. Don't agonize over any other "diet" ever again. Just know what you are electing to do and learn to accept the resulting calamity, which involves misery, disability, discomfort and an earlier than expected death. That sounds harsh, I know, but it's reality. There's no easy way to realize the results you desire.

To achieve outstanding results, people must do what it takes to achieve their goal. Enough said.

What about exercise? Exercise is good, right? Yes, it is, but you are only going to walk for thirty to forty-five minutes per day at least four times per week while undergoing the detoxification process. That's not much, but it's enough for now.

Walking helps move the lymph fluid through the body so it can carry toxins that are hiding in the tissues back to the liver, where they can be metabolized and excreted. Don't exercise more than that regardless of how enthusiastic you are to see the pounds fall off your body.

Strenuous exercise should be put on hold during your detoxification period. Strenuous exercise is undesirable during this time because it will overtax the liver and you don't need that right now. While detoxification is taking place, the liver is in a healing phase, as the Phase I and Phase II excretory pathways are being re-established. This is a bad time to place extra stress on the liver.

Also, strenuous exercise will cause a faster dumping of toxins into the bloodstream as more fat reserves are used up as energy. Remember, most toxins are fat-soluble and are stored by the liver in fatty tissues. If fat reserves are burned up too quickly, toxin levels will skyrocket in your bloodstream, and you will feel awful. This program was designed to be gentle, so don't make it otherwise.

In my *Foods Making You Fat, Unhealthy, and Unhappy: Your Personal Roadmap to Fix Problems Doctors Cannot* book, I explain a plan for you to customize a diet for your body so you can more easily keep the weight off after you've lost it. If you want to lose more weight, simply go back to a detoxification program again. You can continue going back and forth between the detoxification program and the health plan I outline in that book until you reach your desired percentage of body fat. This will allow you to maintain your lowered weight without thinking about it. It's a very cool plan and works exceptionally well for the people who follow it.

Alternating a detoxification program with a healthy eating plan is a reasonable method of losing a lot of weight for the people who have many pounds to shed, and it allows them to do so safely and easily. In this manner, your diet is varied, and not harmfully prohibitive, so weight loss does not become onerous in the least. It is nearly impossible for you to lose large amounts of weight and keep it off if you are required to stay on a rigid or highly restrictive diet for considerable lengths of time. That's the beauty of this process.

The idea is to allow you to establish correct eating habits that result in a healthier weight and make a note of your improved health at the same time. All "diets" you have tried in the past have been much too restrictive and unnatural for your lifestyle. Plus, they did not connect your weight loss with the reduction or disappearance of other symptoms.

That's the beauty of inserting the tenets of behavior modification into the plan as I outline in the book The *Psychology Behind Eating: Scientifically Proven Mind Games to Lose Weight and Keep It Off.* It makes the process stress-free so you can easily stick to the plan for as long as you want to, which should be for life.

So, how are you supposed to take all those nutritional supplements we talked about? Well, it's easy because you don't have to remember anything.

Standard Process packages their detoxification program in a kit with full instructions included. All you must do is follow the directions.

It never fails to amaze me that folks balk at having to take nutritional supplements. Some people have an aversion to "taking all of those pills," even though the supplements are nothing but food! The people who complain about consuming nutritional supplements are usually the same folks taking two handfuls of prescription drugs each day just to stay alive.

Why do they need all those drugs? They need drugs because they refuse to eat healthy foods necessary to maintain a healthy body. Go figure.

Take supplements. They will help make you healthier and slimmer. When your body has the nutrients it needs, it shuts off your "I'm hungry" signals. That's important not only because it will allow you to eat normal amounts of food, but also because it gives your body the nutritional building blocks it needs for normal function. That's very important for your continued wellbeing.

Chapter Thirty-Two

Hallelujah Diet and Lifestyle

Initially, few people are dedicated enough to follow the rigors of this program, but for those who have followed it, the outcomes have been outstanding. However, after consuming a healthier diet for a time and changing your eating habits a bit, you will probably see your food cravings naturally gravitate toward choosing healthier and more nutritious foods. It is at that time you may find yourself more inclined to eat the foods outlined in the Hallelujah Diet.

Your healthier eating habits will spring from eating the foods your body needs and avoiding those it does not want. If you are interested in progressing through the process of making those determinations to fine tune your diet, you will need the additional information found in the other books of the Lose Weight and Regain Health Series.

Having your food cravings change to healthier food choices is a neat thing to see happening, and it does not require huge amounts of willpower. With diligence and eating the foods your body needs, it will evolve on its own.

The Hallelujah Diet has all the facets needed to have a successful liver detoxification experience and to establish positive lifestyle changes. It may be just the ticket for those of you who "want to do it on your own." However, as with any change in eating habits or weight loss program, you should contact your family physician so they know what you are doing and why you are doing it.

The Hallelujah Diet and lifestyle is a Christian influenced diet based upon biblical principles. If this turns you off, just skip to the next section.

If it is interesting to you, then bless you!

The basic premise of the Hallelujah Diet comes from Genesis 1:29, where fresh vegetables, fruits, nuts, and seeds are outlined as the correct way to eat. Look it up for yourself.

I must question why the Hallelujah Diet prohibits meats. After all, Jesus ate fish. Remember the fishes and loaves? Remember when Jesus appeared to His Disciples after His resurrection? He asked for food, and they gave Him fish. And He ate it!

A high-quality source of protein is important to the conjugation process found in Phase II of the liver detoxification process. If you decide to use this plan for detoxification, add a little chicken or fish to it or you will lose muscle mass. You will lose muscle mass if you don't consume protein because your body will break down your own muscles to supply the protein missing from your diet. You do not want that to happen!

The Hallelujah diet may be just fine for a twenty-one-day detoxification program, but it is too restrictive for most of you to follow for any length of time, at least at first. Eventually, your eating habits will change, and you will be better equipped to immerse yourself in this diet.

Raw foods are used on this diet. Cooking foods renders them nutritionally incomplete because heat destroys needed enzymes and nutrients. Raw vegetables supply enzymes and phytonutrients necessary for proper liver function. Do you see a continuing theme here with enzymes and phytonutrients? They're important, so make sure you eat what you need to get them every day.

If you experience detoxification symptoms with this diet, you will know you really needed to be detoxified. Look at the positive long-term benefits. Once you realize that fact, you will better understand and accept why these things are happening. Detoxification symptoms usually only last three to seven days, on average, so just stick with it up and get the job done.

Most toxin elimination takes place through the bowels. Naturally, this is one of the most important aspects of detoxification and must be addressed. If you can't quickly expel toxins, they will have more time to lie in the bowels and be reabsorbed. That's not good.

Prolonged storage of feces in the bowels allows toxins more time to affect the cells of the colon, increasing the potential for colon cancer. That's not good either. Effective bowel function is essential for health. Don't minimize the importance of quickly eliminating waste from your body. Eating a diet high in fiber, along with a lot of water, should take care of any elimination problems you've experienced in the past.

There are some indications that seventy-five to ninety percent of the American public suffers from sluggish bowels. This is not surprising since the typical American diet includes a small amount of bulky fiber and huge amounts of refined foods. Elimination via the bowels must be optimized if you are to achieve true health.

If the bowels are not fully functioning to efficiently eliminate toxins from the body, secondary excretory pathways such as the skin will be pressed into performing these functions. Even the mucous membranes of the sinuses become involved.

I have often thought the mucous membranes become much more sensitive to common items like dust when the liver is overloaded. This may be because the toxins are being expelled via a secondary excretory pathway involving the skin and mucous membranes, increasing their sensitivity.

When people detoxify their liver, many of the "allergies" they had to common environmental irritants suddenly disappear.

It appears the mucous membranes just become more sensitive and react by causing you to sneeze, cough, or have watery eyes. It's not so much a true allergy as it is an irritation to the membranes. Of course, you don't know the difference, you just sneeze your head off.

If these types of symptoms disappear with detoxification, make sure you write it on your "canary" list.

During detoxification, the body may experience flu-like symptoms such as vomiting, depression, headache, fatigue, constipation or diarrhea, fever, skin rashes, irritability, lethargy, and a bunch of other symptoms. Each person's reaction to detoxification is different and covers a wide range of symptoms, or lack of symptoms. Such is life.

Yes, this all sounds bad, but you must remember that detoxification is a positive experience. The benefits far outweigh the potential for temporary discomfort. Of course, that's assuming any detoxification related symptoms occur at all. Often there are none. Let me repeat myself, everyone is different in his or her detoxification experience.

After detoxification, correction of the systems may take up to a year to complete. Therefore, this information should be viewed as a lifestyle change, not a quick fix. This is true for folks constantly being exposed to toxins from within their environment, which, as we have established, is everyone.

However, once the detoxification period is finished, you will feel better than you have in years.

When you are undergoing detoxification, it means your body recognizes things are not right and it is making corrections. The re-establishment of the correct excretory pathways will normalize several bodily functions that have been abnormal for a long time.

The Hallelujah Diet works off an 85%/15% principle. Meaning you eat 85% raw foods and 15% cooked foods. This is often too restrictive for permanent dietary changes and may be too much of a hurtle to overcome for many of you used to the typical American diet.

The 85% portion consists of raw vegetables and supplements. Just make sure you eat raw vegetables for snacks.

Everything taken into consideration, the Hallelujah Diet has some strong points, and it may be just the ticket for you, especially if you add some protein to it.

Which brings us to the third example of liver detoxification. This is a less restrictive program which could be the route you need to take to make a program like this more palatable to you.

Chapter Thirty-Three

Nutri-West Liver Detoxification Program

These products are well known by healthcare professionals and are used with outstanding success by many practitioners, so this approach may be for you.

Is it as good as the other detoxification programs? Is it worse than the others? It's all relative.

By following the Nutri-West detoxification program, you will not lose weight the way you would on the two previously discussed programs unless you eat only vegetables, a little protein in the form of fish or chicken, and fresh fruit. There is no reason you cannot mix-and-match programs and supplements to custom-tailor your own detoxification program.

If you want the ease of taking nutritional supplement pills instead of mixing a "shake" every morning, you can combine the Nutri-West supplements with a vegetable/fruit protocol.

Fruits should still be restricted compared to the number of vegetables you consume daily. If you eat too much fruit in relation to the number of vegetables, you will not lose weight. There is simply too much sugar in fruit and your body will use this high-calorie energy source instead of burning fat.

Vegetables should be the mainstay of your lifestyle-changing program because they supply enzymes and other necessary nutrients you cannot get in other foods, and they are vital to the liver detoxification process. But you will want to avoid eating starchy vegetables like white potatoes, sweet potatoes, pumpkin, corn, green peas, squash, carrots, and parsnips. There are others, but you can research them on the Internet when you are ready.

Remember that you can eat as many fresh vegetables as you can hold because of the vital enzymes and phytonutrients they provide. There is no limit on vegetables. The more the better. Because of the eat-as-many-vegetables-as-you-want facet of liver detoxification and weight loss, you should never go hungry. Ever.

I hope when you begin looking at the consumption of vegetables as being a necessary component of keeping your body healthy instead of something you must do to lose weight it will make it easier for you. Some people are willing to give their body what it needs to remain healthy, and some are not. Keep the enzyme and phytonutrient aspect in mind. It will help get you onto the right path to improving your health.

Fresh fruits you can have include apples, oranges (but not grapefruit because it affects Phase 2 of the detoxification process), bananas, grapes, berries, melons, and tomatoes.

A bit of fish or chicken, about the size of a pack of playing cards, should be consumed every day during any detoxification program. Protein is a necessary component of the detoxification process, so don't forget to include it.

If you detoxify your liver, and then eat any other weight loss "diet" you enjoy, you will have better results on that diet. Use this detoxification information to suit your lifestyle. Just don't expect you can eat anything you want to, in gross amounts, and still lose weight. That just won't happen.

Also, on the Nutri-West program, you will not have stomach shrinking occurring unless you eat a vegetable/fruit protocol. Stomach shrinking is important because the smaller your stomach is, the sooner it will give you the "full" signal telling you to stop eating. By eating a fruit and vegetable protocol for twenty-one days it will help you achieve a smaller, shrunken stomach.

If you do not follow a vegetable/fruit protocol, you will have to exhibit much more willpower when using this less restrictive liver detoxification program. The other two programs, once again, have it built in because they use a vegetable/fruit protocol. Mix-and-match the programs if you want to, see what is agreeable to you and your temperament, and then use it.

This detoxification program entails taking the Nurtri-West product called Total Liver D-Tox. Catchy name, isn't it?

Liver D-Tox will improve the carbohydrate, fat, and protein metabolism functions of the liver. It will also improve the detoxification process, both Phase I and Phase II.

Is this more to your liking? Everything you need in one little nutritional supplement? Handy, eh? But there are more supplements you should be taking during the detoxification phase if you refuse to eat a raw vegetable and fresh fruit protocol.

One product is called Total Veggie. Another really cute name, isn't it? Don't let the charming name fool you though. This stuff is packed with nutrients necessary for improving health.

Total Veggie is full of phytonutrients that are not classified as nutrients yet but have been identified as possessing disease preventative properties. Phytonutrients are involved in preventing cell damage, decreasing cholesterol levels, and helping to protect against other disease processes.

Phytonutrients are found in fresh fruits and vegetables. The consumption of fresh fruits and vegetables has consistently been found to reduce the risk of many degenerative disease processes.

If you opt for this less restrictive liver detoxification program, it may be because you do not have the time or inclination to eat all the raw vegetables you should. Total Veggie will give you just about everything you would get in raw vegetables but in an easy-to-consume form.

Total Veggie is not a perfect substitute for real, organically grown vegetables, but if you will not eat the real thing, for whatever reason, it is better than nothing.

Another Nutri-west product you will want to include in your liver detoxification protocol is Total Trim. No, this is not a "magic diet pill" that will melt fat off you while you sleep like some weight loss products claim. Only fad diets promise to give you something for nothing, and you know that will not happen, right? If fad diets worked as quickly and easily as they proclaim to, why is the incidence of obesity in the United States on the rise? Do yourself a favor and avoid fad diets.

You need balance in your eating habits and life. To do otherwise is to guarantee failure. You will have temporary results and be once again disillusioned by the entire concept of losing weight.

Balancing your diet means consuming the proper ratios of protein, carbohydrates, and fats. These are known as macronutrients. What is important are the types of protein, the type of carbohydrates, and the types of fats that will assist in weight loss then keep that weight off.

Nutritional deficiencies and metabolic problems cause an imbalance in your body that will prevent your ability to achieve balance so weight loss can occur. When your body is deprived of nutrients, it can only create cravings, so you will eat more to secure those missing nutrients.

Concentrated food complexes supply needed nutrients to help reduce your appetite and allow energy expenditures, usually increased through exercise, to burn the stored fat reserves. Eating raw foods as much as possible while avoiding processed foods helps you achieve this goal.

Total Trim has a formula that supports balancing bodily functions and organ systems contributing to the maintenance of a healthier body fat ratio. This includes helping digestion, metabolism, thermogenesis (fat burning), aiding fat mobilization and breakdown, and increasing muscle tone.

Total Trim is a supplement that supports the adrenal glands, thyroid, liver cleansing, and elimination via the colon, all without the use of stimulants such as caffeine or ephedra, which have been shown to be potentially dangerous. Remember, you want to use healthy foods your body needs, not drugs to artificially stimulate weight loss.

By using healthy eating habits, exercising, correcting nutritional deficiencies, and repairing metabolic dysfunction you will aid true weight loss and maintenance for the long term. Naturally, this is not without the potential for problems with some conditions. Total Trim should not be used by phenylketonurics or with MAO inhibitor use. This is where your health care professional's education and guidance will become invaluable to you.

If you opt to use the Nutri-West detoxification program, you should also use a good quality protein drink such as Total Green Protein from that same company. This product has a combination of protein from whey, sprouts, antioxidants, and green vegetables. It supports the protein balance of the body, strengthens the immune system, improves bowel function, and cellular repair. Total Green Protein is also high in fiber and nutrients, which not only suppresses the appetite but also helps to normalize blood sugar.

Using a whey powder like Total Green Protein that supplies protein decreases appetite, thereby reducing caloric intake. Protein powders like this one help the detoxification process by shrinking the caloric load thereby increasing fat burning, which frees toxins so they can be excreted. The nutrients in these powders aid in binding and removing toxins to avoid resorption. By combining the effects of protein with the effects of phytonutrients and fiber, a system for detoxification is established.

Protein powders are easily added to other foods or made into shakes. This is helpful because they lower the glycemic index of carbohydrates if consumed at the same meal. A protein shake consumed between meals helps to stabilize blood sugar, prevent cravings, and alleviate some of your hunger pangs to reduce binge eating until your body stabilizes. Once your body stabilizes and is operating the way it is supposed to, these problems will usually be a thing of the past. Cool, isn't it? If you do right by your body, it will do right by you.

Besides Total Liver D-Tox, Total Trim, Total Green Protein, and Total Veggie (if you want to add it to your regimen to get closer to the daily vegetable intake you should consume) your health care professional may also suggest other Nutri-West products depending on your situation.

For instance, if you suffer from Leaky Gut Syndrome, your health care practitioner may suggest Hypo-D, Total Leaky Gut, or Total Systemic Detox to help with the leaky gut situation. I love those catchy names, don't you?

If stress is increasing your cortisol levels and sabotaging your weight loss efforts, your health care practitioner may suggest Total Cort as a nutritional aid in alleviating this problem.

I always suggest detoxifying your liver first to re-establish its role in cortisol breakdown. This is a more reasonable and successful route to take instead of trying to deal with excessive cortisol production and retention without liver detoxification.

Chapter Thirty-Four

Metagenics Detoxification Program

In the past, I have used Metagenics products with great satisfaction and helped many patients return to health. They are of high quality, work well, and are like the others we've discussed, so we won't waste time going over everything again.

Metagenics offers a detoxification program in addition to gastrointestinal lining support and other wonderful products. You and your healthcare practitioner must determine which is best for you.

Metagenic's UltraClear Plus is the most used product for detoxification. It is often used for people having multiple sensitivities and severe symptoms. This is especially true where multiple symptoms, multiple chemical sensitivities, chronic fatigue syndrome, or fibromyalgia are issues.

You will most likely want to use AdvaClear, a capsule that is formulated for balanced detoxification. It is very important that the detoxification process be balanced; meaning that as Phase I activity is increasing, Phase II activity must also be increasing.

Remember, Phase I creates chemical metabolites that may be very toxic, or even cancer causing, and must be made harmless immediately by being processed through Phase II. You don't want to create a bigger problem without a suitable solution. Phase II must work efficiently if Phase I is producing harmful intermediary chemicals.

There are genuine reasons for eliminating certain food categories from your diet during the Metagenic's detoxification program. These foods will be added back into your diet later in an organized manner so you can monitor any allergy or sensitivity resulting from specific foods.

This is important information for you to understand. It is ludicrous for you to sabotage your health by eating foods you have a food sensitivity to. Your healthcare practitioner is used to working with these types of problems and will be very helpful to you. Use their knowledge and experience to your benefit.

If you want to find any food sensitivities you have on your own, you can learn how to do that in the book *Foods Making You Fat, Unhealthy, and Unhappy: Your Personal Roadmap to Fix Problems Doctors Cannot.* In that book, I go step-by-step through the process of finding your food sensitivities to make it easy for you.

The reality of the situation is that most people have serious nutritional deficiencies and health issues. That's why you are reading this book and is why you're in the shape you're in. If you remember, I said early in this book we would not be looking at weight loss alone. But rather, we will work to restore health to your body and weight loss will follow.

A healthy body is a slim body. And most of you are not healthy, which is why you have an unhealthy accumulation of body fat. As a nation, with the entire world now joining in, people are eating the wrong things. This is detrimental to their health.

Most folks are not interested in "health" because it is a very nebulous term. It's impossible to define exactly what health is, and since it can't be seen, people tend to ignore it. At least until they get seriously ill.

Your healthcare professional, at least the ones that use nutritional counseling and supplementation, truly understands what real health is about. They can offer you information and guidance you will get nowhere else. That's why you should see a healthcare professional to accomplish your goal of weight loss even though you have a ton of information from this book and can do it on your own.

Your healthcare professional has spent literally hundreds of hours and tens of thousands of dollars taking classes, usually after graduating from their professional colleges and universities, to learn the ins and outs of this body of knowledge. They already did extensive research and learned what works and what doesn't, plus, they stay up on the latest data, so you don't have to. Knowledgeable, educated practitioners of the healing arts can guard your safety as they successfully guide you back to true health instead of you needing to spend over eight years of your life in college learning these things.

Some of these detoxification programs are not advertised for weight loss, though that usually occurs if you follow the protocols. However, if you want to lose weight during detoxification, you should work with your healthcare practitioner to develop specific menus and calorie limits that will generate weight loss.

Weight loss usually entails eating only raw vegetables, fresh fruit, and a little protein for the duration of the detoxification process. I understand how daunting this information can be. The detoxification regimen is most likely what your body needs to remove the impediments to you losing weight.

Remember, you can eat anytime you are hungry while on a detoxification plan, if you are eating raw vegetables or fresh fruit. Always remember to stop eating when you are full. I must strongly stress that these two factors are vital to getting you healthier and slimmer and is how you can stay that way.

Chapter Thirty-Five

Detoxification Considerations

It is estimated that many hundreds of billions of dollars are spent in the United States and in Canada each year treating toxicity-related diseases. This statistic must beg the question as to how much of this could be prevented by just eating the correct foods to help the body detoxify toxins naturally.

Toxin exposure has been indicated as causative factors in such diverse health conditions as cancer, atherosclerotic disease (as well as its associated heart disease), diabetes, chronic fatigue syndrome, chemical sensitivity, and even Parkinson's disease.

The statistics regarding cancer alone are staggering with as much as eighty percent of all cancer cases estimated as being environmental toxin related.

Conditions such as brain cancer have increased thirty percent while non-Hodgkin's lymphoma increased twenty-one percent between the years of 1973 and 1997, and that number may have grown since then. A strong correlation exists between these types of cancers and the exposure to organo-chlorinated pesticides. Is this just coincidence? Maybe not.

One of your first lines of defense against environmental toxins may be consuming an adequate amount of dietary fiber daily.

We have discussed the role fiber plays in the detoxification process. Dietary fiber "hides" toxins from the gut wall so they cannot be easily absorbed. It also helps to keep the gut healthy by speeding the movement of food through the intestines, maintaining a healthy acid/base (known as pH) balance in the gut, and assisting bile secretion.

However, all fiber is not created equally. All of it is good, but it's just not all equally good.

While fiber in oats, corn, barley, and wheat can bind toxins and help in their excretion, it is the bran from rice that is particularly good at this function. Note that the bran portion is removed from the polished white rice most often consumed in the United States. Learn to recognize the difference between whole grains and refined grains, as the health ramifications can be significant.

A detailed discussion of whole grains is included in the book *Modified Mediterranean Diet: Your Bridge to a Slimmer, Healthier Body That Looks and Feels Younger.* I give this away for free when people sign up for my email list so make sure you pick up a copy by following the link at the end of this book.

Beneficial fiber consumption is important because most of the conjugated toxins are excreted via the bile. Healthy fecal production, which includes a good source of fiber and adequate water consumption, is essential for efficient expulsion of toxins from your body.

When eating fiber, it is essential to drink plenty, and I mean plenty, of water. Fiber soaks up water like a sponge, which is why you want it in your diet. You need enough water to soak the fiber completely until it cannot absorb any more. Then you need more water to keep the kidneys functioning correctly. You may have to reconsider how much water you are consuming every day and begin forcing yourself to guzzle more.

Remember, toxins are excreted through both the bowels and the kidneys. Both avenues require plenty of water to operate correctly. For some unknown reason, many folks love to brag about how little water they drink each day. I really don't understand how being stupid is anything to brag about.

Many recent reviews of the literature have been able to summarize the current thinking about how you become susceptible to cancer. The most often implicated system protecting you from carcinogens (cancer causing agents) from the environment is the detoxification system.

Regardless of the liver detoxification program you use, consult with a health care professional knowledgeable in this process. If you have an unhealthy accumulation of body fat, you will probably have other health issues that are contributing to your situation.

All aspects of your body are related to many others. If there is a problem with one organ or system, there will be problems with others. Explore all avenues of possible health detriments that may add to your overloaded liver and unhealthy accumulation of body fat. All bodily systems should be normalized if you are to reap the maximum benefit from your detoxification and weight loss endeavors.

Take this to heart. It will not only make you slimmer, but also make you healthier (which makes you look younger and more vibrant). Of course, it can easily be argued that being healthy is much more important than being slim. Really, what good is it doing you to be slim if you're not healthy? You may end up dead before you can make the changes that could have saved your life.

Chapter Thirty-Six

Synopsis for a Slim, Healthy Body

Let's look at a quick summary of the concepts you must follow to gain and maintain a healthy percentage of body fat:

1) Purify and detoxify your liver, then keep it that way (which may involve fixing your Leaky Gut Syndrome first, so it does not continue overloading your liver).

Then all you need to do is take your nutritional supplements and eat enough raw vegetables every day to keep both phases of the liver excretory pathways functioning properly. That's not asking too much, is it?

2) Eat the "good" foods like fresh fruit, raw vegetables, and whole grains to keep you healthy with an appropriate percentage of body fat. It's what your body demands to keep functioning correctly. Give your body what it needs and nothing it doesn't.

3) Take your organically grown whole food nutritional supplements every day to keep your body healthy. It is too hard to regain lost health. This way, you are assured of having the nutritional building blocks your body needs daily without having to think (or worry) about it.

Remember, when your body has all the nutrients it needs at the beginning of your day, it will be satisfied, and your hunger will be lessened.

4) Exercise. Not the sweating and grunting type of exercise. Just get off your posterior and move a little.

5) Monitor your "canaries" weekly and take corrective action if necessary. This is what will help you maintain your weight loss. I address this topic in much more depth in the book *Foods Making You Fat, Unhealthy, and Unhappy: Your Personal Roadmap to Fix Problems Doctors Cannot.*

If you want to maximize your health to its fullest extent, you can read the *Executive Summary and Workbook* which includes all steps I outline to discover how to fine tune your diet so you can discover the foods your body wants and which ones it does not want. Each step in the process takes you deeper into discovering the foods you must avoid based on your unique individual needs.

The *Executive Summary and Workbook* includes an outline of all the steps to fine tune your eating habits as found in all the books in the Lose Weight and Regain Health Series. It is a wonderful resource to use so you are sure to follow the steps in the order they should be used.

Folks with life altering problems like arthritis and other pain syndromes who read the book *Arthritis, Pain Syndromes, and Feeling Older Than You Should: Your Personalized Path to Stop Pain* will need to go from the first step in the process as described in this book and then work their way through all the other steps used to fine tune their eating habits. They will benefit from the outline provided in the *Executive Summary and Workbook* as will the people who simply want to maximize their health, improve how they look, and how they feel.

Readers can stop at any of the steps in the process, but if they are interested in fine tuning their body for maximal benefit, they must go to the end just like the people with arthritis or other pain syndromes. You should take time to look seriously at how your health is being affected by your eating and lifestyle habits. Then take measures to rectify the situation because you may not have a second chance.

A good idea is to read this book again in six months. You will have forgotten much of the information it contains and you will better understand all I was trying to explain.

Also, you will have some experience with all the elements I outlined. A second reading will make much more sense to you, and you will more enthusiastically embrace what it can do for you.

Your health truly is above all gold and treasure. Think about it for a minute and take your health seriously.

You'll be glad you did.

The End

Leave a Review

Please leave a review on Amazon to let other readers know your opinion of this book. It only takes a moment or two by going to:

http://www.amazon.com/review/create-review?&asin=B0BS4JVWYH

Everyone is entitled to their opinion, so please be honest. Your review will mean a lot to future readers. Reviews of books are a vital part of helping readers find books they'll love.

Thank you very much in advance for taking the time to post a review of this book. It is greatly appreciated.

ABOUT THE AUTHOR

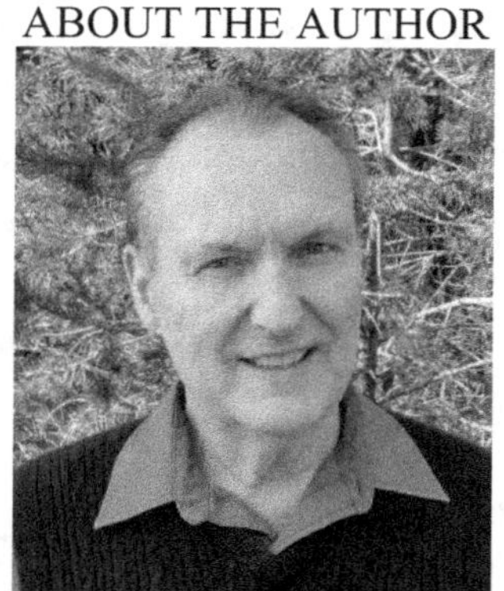

Dr. Heil was born on a wintry day in Pittsburgh in 1956. He received an undergraduate degree in Psychology from Slippery Rock University, spent an adventurous winter in Aspen, CO as a ski bum, then attended the National University of Health Sciences in Lombard, IL where he received a BS in Human Biology and a Doctorate in Chiropractic.

In addition to writing fiction as well as non-fiction books, Dr. Heil recently obtained a Master's degree in Industrial and Organizational Psychology.

He and his wife live in Pennsylvania where they raised their four children.

Do You Like Suspense Thrillers?

If so, check out some of Dr. Heil's by going to www.DEHeil.com

There are a few thriller books there you can try for FREE.

The Psychology Behind Eating:

Scientifically Proven Mind Games to Lose Weight and Keep It Off

Book Two of the Lose Weight and Regain Health Series

Dr. Dale Heil

Receive a FREE Gift!

Building a relationship with my readers is the absolute best thing about writing. I love to send newsletters with details on new releases, special offers, and other bits related to the Lose Weight and Regain Health Series so we can build that relationship.

Get a FREE copy with email signup of the eBook *Modified Mediterranean Diet: Your Bridge to a Slimmer, Healthier Body That Looks and Feels Younger* by going to:

https://dl.bookfunnel.com/2b7k9uiilq

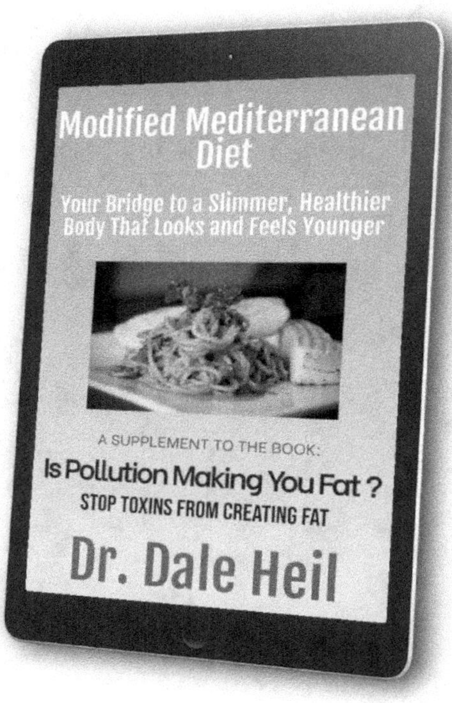

Chapter 1

Setting The Stage for Learning

In the first book of this series, *Is Pollution Making You Fat? Stop Toxins from Creating Fat* we showed how environmental pollution and toxins overload the liver, establishing vicious cycles of fat production and how to cure this situation. Now, let's look at how psychology can help you get on the right track to not only lose weight or stay healthy, depending on what your goals are (it could be both), but also assure that you stay that way for the rest of your life.

Why is psychology important? Well, let's explore that for a moment.

We've all heard about people who go on a diet, lose a lot of weight, and feel great, but before they know it, they've gained all their weight back plus a few pounds along with their health robbing symptoms. If you're reading this book, you may have experienced that a time or two (or ten, if you are truthful with yourself). Most people have.

The reason you will fail almost every time you try going this route is that you did not know how to apply the simple principles of behavior modification to what you want to accomplish... and you're also most likely eating the wrong foods to lose weight or stay healthy.

This has little to do with the factors making you fat, like we discussed in the first book. It has everything to do with you not understanding how certain foods react with your body.

Since you are now reading the second book in this book series, let me explain how I organized this information. The first book in the series showed people how to stop the formation of vicious cycles of fat production so they can lose weight.

This second book of the series about psychology is necessary because our mind dictates how successful we will be with losing weight and then keeping it off. Why lose all that weight just to put it all back on again? It's what usually happens with people's weight loss efforts, and I wrote this book to avoid that from happening to you.

The third book of the series is entitled *Foods Making You Fat, Unhealthy, and Unhappy: Your Personal Roadmap to Fix Problems Doctors Cannot.* If your goal is only to lose weight and keep it off, the first two books are enough for you. I wrote this third book for people who want to be as healthy as they can be, or those who have terrible health problems they want to reduce or even eliminate.

The fourth book of the series is for people who have very serious health issues that are gravely affecting their lives. It is called *Arthritis, Pain Syndromes, and Feeling Older Than You Should: Your Personalized Path to Stop Pain.*

Each of these books takes the reader further into determining which foods they should eat, and which ones are detrimental to their health. I wrote them in a series because everyone may not want to follow the process to the end because they are happy stopping somewhere along the way. By setting this book series up in this manner, readers can get the results they crave and stop when they want to.

In this book on the psychology of eating, I will teach you how to use simple principles of behavior modification to change your eating habits permanently in an easy to learn step-by-step strategy so you can effortlessly manage food and its effect on your life. To begin this discussion of how to use psychology to make your journey toward a slimmer, healthier body an easier one, let's look at children and the problems they have with carrying an abnormal amount of body fat.

But why should we look at the eating habits of children? Why not get straight to the good stuff about psychology and how you can use it to get your slimmer, healthier body? Simple. It's because the eating habits you developed as a child shaped your eating habits as an adult. How did you learn those eating habits? Your parents and peers taught them to you. Just like a baby bird learns to eat worms because that's what momma bird and daddy bird taught them to eat, you learned your eating habits from your parents and friends.

Kids learn by watching others, which is most often their parents in their early years. The psychology that went on during your formative years has shaped you in ways you cannot imagine. As we progress through this discussion about children, see if a lot of it doesn't remind you of your upbringing.

***

Continue reading the second book of this series, *The Psychology Behind Eating: Scientifically Proven Mind Games to Lose Weight and Keep It Off* by going to:

https://amzn.to/3XUE9eA

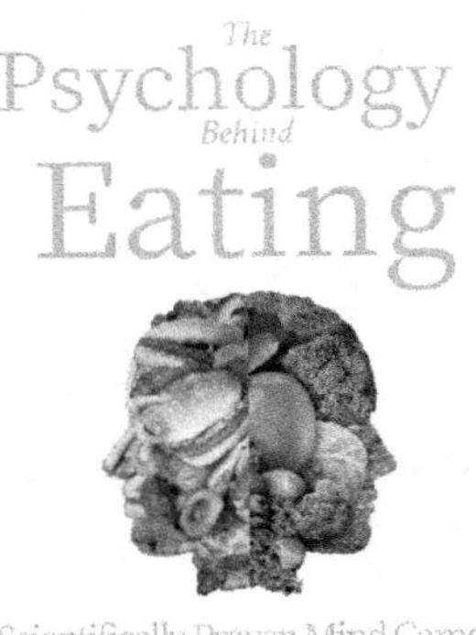